Dyslexia

Dyslexia

The Government of Reading

Tom Campbell
University of Leeds

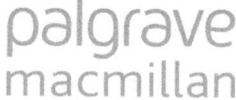

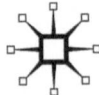

First published 2013 by
PALGRAVE MACMILLAN

Palgrave Macmillan in the UK is an imprint of Macmillan Publishers Limited, registered in England, company number 785998, of Houndmills, Basingstoke, Hampshire RG21 6XS.

Palgrave Macmillan in the US is a division of St Martin's Press LLC, 175 Fifth Avenue, New York, NY 10010.

Palgrave Macmillan is the global academic imprint of the above companies and has companies and representatives throughout the world.

Palgrave® and Macmillan® are registered trademarks in the United States, the United Kingdom, Europe and other countries

ISBN: 978–1–137–29792–1

This book is printed on paper suitable for recycling and made from fully managed and sustained forest sources. Logging, pulping and manufacturing processes are expected to conform to the environmental regulations of the country of origin.

A catalogue record for this book is available from the British Library.

A catalogue record for this book is available from the Library of Congress.

Contents

Acknowledgements

My mother and father, June and Simon, must be thanked first for their unwavering belief and limitless support throughout my education. Without this support, particularly in my formative years (where they fought for me tirelessly), I would not have had the opportunity to write this book. Similarly, there can be no doubt that Amy Charlesworth's intellectual support throughout was invaluable in bringing this project to fruition, and that says nothing of the proofing of draft after draft, and constant encouragement.

I would like to thank all my colleagues, past and present, at the School of Sociology and Social Policy, University of Leeds, UK. In particular, Mark Priestley and Anne Kerr, whose careful mentoring added much to the project and my intellectual development. Conversations with Chris Till, Mark Davis, Paul Bagguley, Angharad Beckett and Austin Harrington have all, in different ways, shaped the character of the book. I also thank the staff and students of the Department of Disability and Human Development, University of Illinois, Chicago, IL, USA, where much of the research for this book was completed, for welcoming me.

Various friends and colleagues have looked over earlier drafts, and I would like to extend my gratitude to them all, but particular appreciation is owed to Ben, who read the final manuscript.

An earlier version of Chapter 4 appears in Health Sociology Review (2011), 20(4), 450–61.

1
Introduction

The diagnosis of 'dyslexia' and the medical problematisation of reading difficulties were almost unknown 100 years ago, yet today the British Dyslexia Association (2010) estimates that up to 10% of the UK population may have some form of dyslexia; in the USA it is estimated to be as much as 20% of the population (Marazzi, 2011a). The first diagnosis of dyslexia-like symptoms as a congenital impairment was recorded in Morgan's (1896) paper in the *British Medical Journal*, 'A Case of Congenital Word Blindness'. At the turn of the twentieth century five people had been diagnosed as dyslexic; at the turn of the twenty-first century, the Dyslexia Institute estimated that there are six million individuals who could be diagnosed with some form of dyslexia in the UK alone.[1] At the turn of the twentieth century, fewer than ten articles had been published on reading disabilities, yet today a search for dyslexia on *Google Scholar* returns 120,000 entries. With this rapid growth in numbers of diagnoses and the proliferation of pages written on this topic, it is no surprise that in the middle of the twentieth century dyslexia was proclaimed to be the disease of the century (Mucchielli, 1963). Throughout the twentieth century, laboring began to increasingly rely upon our linguistic and communicative capacities. Literacy became central to production, and dyslexia came to describe a difficultly with a key characteristic of the newly dominant style of laboring in the West.

The research problem I wish to investigate is how, over a relatively short period of time, this newly-diagnosed impairment has become so ubiquitous, and ask how such a diagnosis becomes legitimate as a significant psycho-medical category. Using the example of dyslexia, this book investigates which political, economic and moral forces are involved in the formation of a diagnostic category; how new categories of medical, psychological and administrative labelling are formed; what

1

factors contribute to their invention; and how diagnostic discourses are legitimised through legislative change, educational policy and the practices—discursive and otherwise—of educational psychologists, teachers and parliamentarians. The genealogy of the diagnostic category that is drawn within these pages begins with the first murmurings around its invention, taking in its ossification and eventual diffusion into a variety of different disciplinary fields.

The primary objective of this book is to examine the social relations that allowed the diagnostic category of dyslexia to form. Through historical scholarship it aims to show *how* this happened—through an analysis and description of this material, assertions are made about *why* this diagnostic category was invented. This investigation is primarily concerned with trying to explain why industrialising societies began to regard certain previously invisible phenomena, or unproblematic characteristics, as impairments. Various different vocabularies have been deployed to describe the symptoms that will become understood as dyslexia. The first was 'congenital word-blindness'. Others deployed at various points in time include 'congenital aphasia', 'alexia', 'symbol amblyopia' and 'amnesia visualis verbalis'.

As the pages that follow are mainly concerned with the formation of an obscure medical diagnosis (congenital word-blindness) over a century ago, it may seem to the reader that this investigation is an impersonal endeavour concerned with small events in the annals of the history of medicine. The problems that I am investigating are, in fact, deeply personal; it is an attempt to understand my own relationship with a diagnosis I received as a 10-year-old—a diagnosis that, once received, enabled me to access support that changed my educational experiences. The writing of this book was ultimately motivated by a desire to understand *how* it has become possible for me (and others like me) to receive such a diagnosis. This question has its origins through a reading of two literatures: the philosophy of Michel Foucault and disability studies. I became convinced that disability should be understood as a social phenomenon and, concurrently, that the historical formation of the categories we use to describe ourselves should be carried out to produce, as Foucault has suggested, an ontology of ourselves. Tracing the genealogy of dyslexia became the object of my research, and my investigations were aimed toward understanding how a proliferation of impairment categories across the twentieth century shifted the way that we think of our own bodies and the bodies of others.

Further elaboration on the way so-called Foucauldian genealogy has been operationalised in this book is provided below, but first I would like to draw attention to a key distinction between this book and previous genealogies—the specificity and size of the object in question. Foucault's most famous genealogies deal with modern forms of punishment and sexuality, while other influential studies deal with disciplines such as psychology, as detailed by Nikolas Rose's work or Ian Hacking's work on statistics. The object of my research is undoubtedly more modest, with dyslexia being a single psycho-medical diagnosis rather than a large and pervasive discipline. Treating psycho-medical categories as technologies of power has particular analytical advantages. Unlike Foucault-inspired histories of disability, such as Henri Jacques Stiker's genealogies of impairment categories, will contribute toward to the historical understanding of disability not through analysing disability as a totality but, instead, through describing the conditions of possibility for a specific impairment category the rationale behind why particular human characteristics are problematised will be mapped.

This study, therefore, is a response to calls for a sociology of impairment, but does not respond to these calls by developing a sociology of impairment that focuses on lived experience or embodiment. Rather, varied genealogies of impairment categories are proposed, which are able to describe the conditions that problematise specific human attributes. This study is one such genealogy. Diagnostic and impairment categories alike are to be understood as technologies of power whose workings and operations can be mapped. The second advantage is that unlike those genealogies that describe the operation of power at the level of the individual and the population, genealogies of impairment categories are able to describe how the constitution of the body and the population, through the prism of bio-politics, makes it possible for power to flow at both molecular and molar levels. Genealogies of impairment categories therefore form a necessary appendage to the various genealogies of scientific disciplines (Hacking, 1982, 1990, 1991; Miller, 1992; Rose 1985, 1999) that have corrected and deepened our understanding of the shift from sovereign power to bio-power.[2] The appendage offered hopes to augment the detail by which we can understand the modulation of power, as it infuses and traverses across institutions, machineries of government and the body of the population. How power becomes entwined with capital, coming to act in a molecular fashion, on diverse human characteristics is beyond the vision of the human eye. The individual body is replaced as the object of tactics of power, as discrete and distinct attributes become open to management. It is hoped that these genealogies, focused upon a smaller object of inquiry, will allow for an analytical contribution to the understanding of power that enriches, rather than repeats, Foucault's thesis of the shift from sovereign power to bio-power.

Christian Marazzi's analysis of post-Fordism suggests that this economic shift can, perhaps, be understood as a linguistic turn in the economy (Marazzi, 2011b; Marazzi et al., 2008). This builds on the work from those involved in the *Operaismo* and *Autonomia* movements, particularly the research conducted on immaterial labour, cognitive labour and the increasing deployment of our general linguistic capacity in contemporary forms of capitalist production. His writing draws attention to the relationship between financialisation and language; to the increasing articulation of our general linguistic capacity into production; to the way in which the capitalist mode of production itself becomes, in many ways, a language. Aphasia and dyslexia are explored by these writers to help describe the conditions experienced by the cognitive worker in contemporary capitalism (Lotringer and Marazzi, 2007). Paolo Virno (2003) fired the first salvo, relating how our general linguistic capacity has become the very point upon which contemporary immaterial exploitation is built. Even in successful communication, something remains unrealisable and opaque. For Virno, this is a kind of aphasia and, as such, it is a site that should be defended against commodification and exploitation. Franco 'Bifo' Berardi points to the 'dizzying' rise of dyslexia in the youngest generations, particularly 'in the social and professional classes most involved in the new technologies of communication' (Berardi, 2009: 87) The acceleration of labouring under cognitive capitalism means we not only do not have the time to read a page from beginning to end, but that we are also becoming increasingly incapable of doing so. Marazzi (2011a), points to the importance of understanding dyslexia for analysing the dynamics of cognitive capitalism. In his account, the number of diagnoses has grown over the last 30 years in conjunction with the linguistic turn in the economy. Alberto Toscano (2008) provides a concise summary of this analysis:

> In a recent investigation into managerial thinking on the virtues of dyslexia, Christian Marazzi has pointed to the manner in which the informational saturation-bombing and 'anthropological shock' that characterises contemporary financialised capitalism has turned a linguistic pathology into a subjective 'comparative advantage'. Fortune 500, among others, has honed in on 'dyslexic achievers' as a category of managers, who mine their condition for the 'capacity to alter and create perceptions, an extreme awareness of the environment

in which one is immersed, a greater-than-average curiosity, an ability to think in images, intuition and introspection, multi-dimensional thinking and perception, a capacity of feeling thought as real, a vivid imagination'. (2008: 67)

The importance placed by autonomist thinkers on the diagnosis of dyslexia for understanding the cognitive character of contemporary capitalism suggests that it is particularly indicative of the contemporary conditions of laboring. Marazzi (2011a; Marazzi et al., 2008) has been concerned with theorising how an economic shift—from Fordism to post-Fordism—re-constituted a linguistic pathology into a comparative advantage. In this book, however, I describe the process by which these characteristics became understood as a linguistic pathology. I hope to underline how the organisation of an economy and a style of government can produce impairment categories. Mapping the conditions of diagnostic possibility will indicate the conditions in the mode of production and rationalities of government that have augmented human labour as power is increasingly directed towards the utilisation of our general linguistic capacity. The diagnosis of dyslexia points towards the productive nature of knowledge existing between us, in the commons. Language has often been understood as the key mechanism for understanding the common character of production or, more precisely, how production can have a common character; the diagnosis of dyslexia seems to suggest that mechanisms, for instance the printed page or a tablet screen, through which we access knowledge produce barriers that make it difficult for some people to access the material upon which collective production depends.

The formation of diagnostic categories to describe specific learning difficulties suggests an anthropological shift that proceeds Marazzi's 'anthropological shock'. A shift that, in my view, is best understood through the intersection of two lines. The first is that immaterial or cognitive labour has significantly increased its importance in the character of our economy, resulting in specific problematisations of human flesh, whereby characteristics that were previously unproblematic become pathologised; as the bodies most hospitable to the accumulation of capital are transformed; and as our linguistic capacity becomes increasingly articulated into the accumulation of capital. The second traces the manner in which power operates upon both the body of the individual and the body of the population. By flowing onto increasingly microscopic sites, power can act upon a layer of human flesh that is invisible to the naked eye. In contemporary capitalism the diagram of the human that power is able to operate on 'is man plotted by a thousand numbers'—a plotting that makes possible a diagram where we can be understood as thousands upon thousands of spectrums, dots on lines, that can be acted upon, cultivated and manipulated. Through writing a genealogy of dyslexia I hope to illuminate the way in which the diagram of the body moves from being material to immaterial as it takes on a microscopic and panoramic view simultaneously. Out of this diagrammatic shift developed an array of techniques and practices that can act upon attributes beyond the body visible to human eyes, beyond the touch of human hands. This discussion is taken forward in Chapters 2 and 3.

Investigating the genealogy of dyslexia will contribute to understanding this shift for two key reasons. First, like all impairment categories, it is a technology of power that, when engaged to accredit an individual as dyslexic, also serves to carve a population from the multitude—a population of dyslexics. The diagnosis is both a consequence of and contributing factor to the increasing de-materialisation of the figure of the human. Second, the diagnosis itself describes a difficulty with an activity of immaterial labour—reading. The diagnosis makes possible the management of bodies engaged in immaterial labour. Investigating the conditions that made it possible to diagnose an individual as dyslexic and the way the diagnosis operates as a technology of power will provide a better understanding of the workings of a post-Fordist mode of production wherein immaterial labour has become increasingly commonplace. It is, of course, not surprising that as a linguistic capacity becomes increasingly articulated into the character of labour, a diagnosis that identifies a perceived pathology in one's linguistic capacity would see a growth in the frequency of its diagnosis.

This study hopes to enrich the Foucauldian understanding of the shift from sovereign power to bio-power by illustrating how the constitution of the two-headed body—the individual and the population—also had the effect of producing a new diagram of the human. A diagram that, in it's mapping of human flesh, went beyond the capabilities of the human eye producing a variety of technical devices to view bodies through making visible a field that was simultaneously microscopic and panoramic in its character; a field of vision that made possible the 'the plotting of man by a thousand numbers'. If Nikolas Rose, Ian Hacking, Peter Miller and others have augmented Foucault's understanding of the shift from sovereign power to bio-power by providing further historical evidence for a shift in the style of government, then this study intends to focus upon a diagnostic category that is made possible by the emergent diagram of man. A re-imagining of human flesh that can occur after the diagram of the human begins a process of immaterialisation.

The research that develops from these concerns will endeavor to identify the political, economic and historical reasons *why* dyslexia emerged as a potential area of investigation, and *how* the diagnostic category of dyslexia became legitimised over the course of the twentieth century; how it became entwined with the rise of a new industry of educational psychologists and educationalists geared towards identifying dyslexics and providing for their needs. This is a historical study that investigates how the problematisation of a particular set of characteristics took place and how this became legitimised through disciplinary practices. To address these wider concerns the following specific questions will underpin the discussion that follows in the forthcoming chapters.

- How did it become possible to diagnose congenital reading disabilities from the 1890s onwards?
- What socio-economic, legislative and policy developments can be linked to the formation and development of such diagnoses? For instance, did the introduction of compulsory education from the 1870s onwards, or the emergence of a knowledge economy, help to establish the conditions of possibility that facilitated the diagnosis's formation?
- Did the diagnosis of dyslexia as we know it today develop from a single category, or did it develop as different administrative, medical, psychological and educational categories. Moreover, do different groups utilise different definitions of the same 'diagnosis'?
- How did the different groups who deployed this diagnosis category interact; did they clash or compromise, or was a consensus achieved?

The strategy that has been developed to answer these questions utilises a wide variety of documents to analyse the relations of power that have crafted our bodies, describing the political, economic and technological rationalities that entwined to form particular practices and values. A particular elaboration of this strategy is provided later, in the section entitled 'Genealogy'. Studies of bio-politics and work using a genealogical method are deployed to aide the description of how the characteristics that the diagnosis of dyslexia illuminates became problematised by particular social, technological, economic and political processes. The discussion of these accounts allows the description of relations of power that is advanced within these pages to take on a diagonal character, as dyslexia is situated, as a component, or perhaps a cog, in a machinery of government concerned with performing a multifarious array of operations.

My research problem developed out of an engagement with Foucault's historical studies on the one hand and questions that were being raised through my engagement with disability studies on the other. A number of historical studies that have drawn extensively on Foucault have also be mined for methodological insights, concepts and historical analysis. From reading this literature it became apparent that a shift in the style of government[3] and the rising prestige of disciplines like psychology and the invention of technologies like the norm were events that may have facilitated the invention of dyslexia as a diagnostic device. I have attempted to synthesise the arguments made in a variety of these studies to provide a background for events that were taking place during this period that I think are particularly pertinent to the development of dyslexia as a technology of power.[4] To describe the conditions that shaped dyslexia as a technology of power, and the operation that this technology is able to perform, I have turned to Foucault's genealogical method, which requires some specific and detailed explanation.

Genealogy

Foucault's genealogies surpassed those of Friedrich Nietzsche, at least in one respect: their level of historical scholarship and their more specific focus. Foucault utilises documentary material in a more rigorous fashion than Nietzsche. His studies are more thorough and considerably longer, relying upon a large body of archival material. In Foucault's genealogies the analysis of moral concepts is developed into the description of the strategic utilisation of power, as moral concepts come to be understood as technologies utilised to conduct the conduct of others. While Nietzsche spent an aphorism analysing the morality of punishment, Foucault makes this a book-length study (1977) with supporting lectures, interviews and political activity [see Foucault's involvement with his *Groupe d'information sur les Prisons* (Miller, 1993) or the lectures at *College de France* (Foucault, 2003, 2006b)]. The formation of moral concepts in Foucault's work becomes an analysis of how relations of power came to configure particular moral values, and how moral values came to operate upon bodies. How strange accidents—the collision of a variety of technologies of power and purposeful strategies of government—coalesce to produce particular moral values. For instance, in the opening pages of *Discipline and Punish* two distinct strategies for punishing criminals, with a variety of morals attached to them, are juxtaposed and described as different, but strangely similar, in the way they ultimately act upon the body of the condemned (1991: 3–7). Foucault's genealogy is a scholarly activity concerned with re-problematisation. Restoring histories to objects, where their pasts, as a series of events, had been mystified (Foucault, 2000b: 223–9); this is the methodological line I have attempted to follow, by describing the forces—be they political, technical or economic—that facilitated the formation of the diagnostic category dyslexia.

The commitment to the analysis of the present (Foucault, 1997a, 2010) found in the genealogical tradition is derived from a view of our current world as somewhat arbitrary (Deleuze, 1986: 27–9). Things could always have been different. As with Klossowski (2000) and Deleuze's (1986) categorisation of Nietzsche's thought as returning chance to history, genealogy aims to disturb the ahistorical character of the present. Events have not unfolded in a predetermined order, but have been influenced by accidents, manipulation and the interactions of different strategies of government (Foucault, 1998a). The genealogist believes that if the past was not fixed, then the future is not always as fixed as it may seem (Rose, 1999: xii). Genealogical investigations reveal how relations of power coalesced, in what were then often peculiar and unstable fashions, to form objects—now considered to be immobile, without a history—to be beyond political influence and without a strategic function (Foucault, 1998a, 2000a: 375). The knowledge a genealogist generates is not made for 'knowing', but for cutting. It cuts away at the formations of power and knowledge that have come to be seen as timeless, natural or as bearing a political purpose that has becomes less visible (Foucault, 2000a: 380).

As the present is characterised as a series of events (Foucault, 2000b: 223–9), genealogists have a particular distaste for the conception of the present as a high-point or completion (Foucault, 2000c: 450) This distaste was shared with the prominent French Nietzscheans that Foucault aligned himself with, namely Deleuze (1986) and Klossowski (2000):

> ...one of the harmful habits contemporary thought, in modern thought; even; at any rate in post-Hegelian thought: the analysis of the present as being precisely, in history, a present rupture, of high point, of completion of a returning dawn, etc. (Foucault, 1998b: 450)

The genealogist tries to reinstate our knowledge of how particular machineries of government have been constituted by particular relations of power, by competing rationalities and strategies of government. The genealogist is writing against the idea of the present as a high point, an inventible point of completion. If psychiatry is the object of study for the genealogist (Rose, 1985: 19), it is not the intention to prove that psychiatry does not work. A genealogy does not, indeed, undermine the utility of an endeavour, but aims to describe the strategic games and relations of power that took place around its invention and development—relations of power that in some cases have become invisible (Foucault, 2000b: 226).

For a genealogist, knowledge is an event. This means that when attempting to restore the status of an object such as sexuality to an event in the past one also restores the status of the event to the object in question in the present. Genealogists are attempting to remind their readers that they can still take part in 'inventing' the object; it's ossification, despite appearances, is never complete. The genealogist derives hope from dynamic human life, affirming that stasis is a mystification. Against the mystification of stasis, the genealogist affirms, joyfully, *life* as a process. Once its epistemological status as an event is restored (Foucault, 2000a: 15), possible futures will appear less fixed. Re-situating the object of this study, the diagnosis of dyslexia, as an event, involves mapping the relations of power that led to the problematisation of the characteristics the diagnosis describes.

There are always relations of power running behind and through knowledge. Relations of power that form a complex strategic matrix, that allow for particular phrases to be spoken or for particular practices to appear logical. The activity of genealogy uses documents to attempt to describe the battles that were incurred over particular formations of power and knowledge. By attempting to trace these battles between various experts the particular strategic character of a discursive formation often becomes clear. The matrix of power relations can then be described in a diagrammatic fashion (Deleuze, 1992), for instance Foucault's Panopticon in *Discipline and Punish* (1977) or the line drawn from the confessional pew to the psychiatrist's couch in the first volume of *The History of Sexuality* (1979). The primary diagram that shall be described herein is the gaining of jurisdiction over reading difficulties by psychology and a loss of jurisdiction by ophthalmology, which came to look like a conflict between two strategies concerned with how to govern a population. I have attempted to describe this transformation diagrammatically by sketching the relations of power that facilitated the formation of dyslexia as a diagnostic category and to outline the way that dyslexia as a technology of power allows relations of power to flow onto bodies. The mapping of this diagram aims to contribute to the cartography of a broader shift in the style of government; describing how, over the course of the twentieth and twenty-first centuries, the image of the individual and the population becomes increasingly microscopic and panoramic as the entwined forces of bio-power and capital came to act on our most minute of attributes, and as our general linguistic capacity was articulated into the manner in which human labour power was deployed.

A genealogist approaches the mapping of a strategy of government by

> ...a refusal of analyses couched in terms of the symbolic field or the domain of signifying structures, and a recourse to analyses in terms of the genealogy of relations of force, strategic developments, and tactics...The history which determines us has the form of a war rather than that of language: relations of power, not relations of meaning. (Foucault, 1980: 114)

Studies conducted from the genealogical perspective attempt to outline 'the political and economic conditions of existence that are not a veil or an obstacle for the subject of knowledge but the means by which subjects of knowledge are formed, and hence are truth relations' (Foucault, 2000a: 15). This opposes some notions of ideology where 'ideology is a sort of negative element through which the fact is conveyed that the subject's relation to truth, or simply the knowledge relation, is clouded, obscured, violated by conditions of existence, social relations, or the political forms imposed on the subject of knowledge form the outside' (Foucault, 2000a: 15). Strategic relations of power and economic circumstance do not hide truth; they do not efface the real. Economic circumstance and relations of power constitute truth. They produce reality (Foucault, 1977: 194).

When Foucault writes about Nietzsche's writings on history and truth he pays close attention to the words used by Nietzsche to describe invention (2000a). He returns to the German stating that the words *Erfindung* (invention) and *Ursprung* (origin) are juxtaposed in Nietzsche (1998). This is because human hands have made things. They do not emerge completed, with a destiny already set. For Foucault, following Nietzsche, moral values have been invented by humans, fashioned by human hands, rather than having a divine or otherworldly origin (2000a: 7–15). Using the term invention also suggests that the formation was a process that could have involved detailed plans, arbitrary accidents and may have become a successful invention because of its political merit (Foucault, 1998a). As Foucault states on Nietzsche's examples of religion and poetry:

> Religion has no origin, it has no *Ursprung*, it was invented, there was an *Erfindung* of religion. At a particular moment in the past, something happened that made religion appear. Religion was made; it did not exist before ... Speaking of poetry, still in The Gay Science, Nietzsche declares that: there are those who look for the origin, the *Ursprung*, of poetry, when in fact there is no *Ursprung* of poetry, there is no invention of poetry. Somebody had the rather curious idea of fusing a certain number of rhythmic or musical properties of language to speak, to impose his words, to establish by means of those words a relation of power over others. Poetry, too, was invented or made. (2000a: 7)

In my attempt to write a genealogy of dyslexia, I have not attempted the search for an origin for diagnosis, preferring to try to describe its invention. At a practical level this results in dyslexia being treated as an event or, indeed, as a series of events. In my research (Foucault, 2000a: 15, 2000b: 223–9) I have not searched for a fully constituted diagnosis, but have tried to record the events by which the diagnostic categories developed, in some cases disappeared or ossified. Events are, of course, affected by a wide variety of external factors and genealogy uses documents to try and describe these events.

A Restorative Practice

Genealogy is a restorative practice that aims to reinstate an object with the status of being an event. This is distinct from announcing that the object under investigation was socially constructed, as

> Objects of thought are constructed in thought: what else could they be? So the interesting questions concern the ways in which they are constructed. Where do objects emerge? Which are the authorities which are to pronounce upon them? Through what concepts and explanatory regimes are they specified? How do certain constructions acquire the status of truth—through experimental procedures demonstrations and other inventions, through the production of effects and the reflection on effects, through the rhetorical deployment of evidence and logic and so forth? (Rose, 1999: xi)

What the genealogist is studying is the textual traces of the invention of the object under investigation, the processes and events that were related to its legitimisation. To do this genealogy must 'describe the material and practical conditions under which truths, facts, explanations come to be formulated and accepted and to examine their consequences—what they make possible' (Rose, 1999: xiv). To do this the genealogist must describe the relations between discursive and non-discursive formations.

Discursive formations are made up of statements (Foucault, 1989a: 127). Discourses are not found in isolation, but rather make up formations that rely upon one another for their grounding (Hook, 2001: 33). These discourses are interconnected, and interdependent; there is no such thing as an isolated discourse. Discourses are always discursive formations, interdependent and entwined with one another (Henriques, 1984: 106). The statement's relation to a discursive formation is established by Foucault:

> A statement belongs to a discursive formations as a sentence belongs to a text, and a proposition to deductive whole. But whereas the regularity of a sentence is defined by the laws of language (langue), and that of a proposition by the laws of logic, the regularity of statements is defined by the discursive formation itself. The fact its belonging to a discursive formation and the laws that govern it are one and the same thing; this is not paradoxical since the discursive formation is characterized not by principles of construction but by a desperation of fact, since for statements it is not a condition of possibility but a law of coexistence, and since statements are not interchangeable elements but groups characterized by their modality of existence. (1989a: 130–1)

A discursive formation limits what can be enunciated in a particular statement. Deleuze describes the role that Foucault gives the various discursive formations of medicine as 'Each historical medical formation modulated a first light and constituted a space of visibility for illness, making symptoms gleam' (1992: 58). The role that these discourse formations have for Deleuze is to illuminate particular characteristics. They establish in the case of a disease what symptoms shall be the most prominent in the diagnosis. Deleuze's discourses imbue phenomena with light that makes them visible. Discursive formations, for instance, establish the rules that are necessary for a disease to be accepted. My study is concerned with describing the process that casts light onto the characteristics that are now described as the psycho-medical diagnosis of dyslexia.

The discursive formations that I am studying are not ideas, but practices (Kendal and Wickham, 1999: 42). According to this approach all practices studied by genealogy are 'by definition both discursive and material' (Henriques, 1984: 106) in that they are accessed through textual inscriptions, but are chosen because they are run through with relations of power and are directed towards bodies (Deleuze, 1992: 16). The discursive practices that are being studied are textual records of plans for strategies of government, or records of activities of government. This makes the genealogical study of discourses distinct from the history of ideas, as it is concerned with how people were acted upon (Miller and Rose, 1990). Genealogy tries to describe how discourses become connected to bodies, how they are inserted into machineries of government and how they exist interdependently with relations of power. The genealogical study of discursive practices eschews transcendental analysis where discourses are conceived of as floating above society in some fashion. Discursive formations are to be analysed as interdependent with non-discursive formations and relations of power (Henriques, 1984: 106).

The statements chosen to be analysed in my study will deploy the same criteria as recognised by Deleuze: 'the words phrases and propositions examined by the text must be those which revolve round different focal points of power (and resistance) set in play by a particular problem' (Deleuze, 1992: 16). Klossowksi makes a related point describing how Nietzsche's analyses were concerned with the body (2000: 30). Genealogy has operationalised this by focusing on how the body is operated on by discursive formations and the relations of power running through them.

The description of statements that are clustered around focal points of power and resistance means that genealogy moves from the study of discursive formations to describing the relation between discursive and non-discursive formations. Non-discursive formations include political events, economic processes and institutions (Deleuze, 1992: 9). This relationship between discursive and non-discursive formations is illustrated well by Foucault:

> ...it was political practice that from the early nineteenth century imposed on medicine such new objects as tissular lesions or the antomo-physiological correlations; but it opened up new fields for the mapping of medical objects ([...] the mass of the population

administratively compartmented and supervised [...] the great con-script armies [...] the institution of hospital assistance that were defined at the end of the nineteenth centuries, in relation to the eco-nomic needs of the time and to the reciprocal position of the social classes). One can also see the appearance of this relation of political practice to medical discourse in the status accorded to the doctor... (quoted in Deleuze, 1992: 10)

Institutions imply the existence of statements, charters, contracts, reg-istrations and enrolments. Statements also refer to the institutional cir-cumstances in which they are formed (Deleuze, 1992: 9). It is this relation that genealogy seeks to describe. Through utilising the rules proposed by Kendal and Wickham (1999: 42) I have attempted to describe how the regularity of a discursive formation is affected by non-discursive formations, and the functions that statements perform for particular institutions. Through this method I will be able to describe the central object of my investigations: understanding dyslexia as a technology— a technology of power—and the rationalities that animate its opera-tion. The concept of 'technology' is being deployed with a Foucaulidan inflection; a discussion of the use of this concept throughout this book is provided in Chapter 3, 'Governing Readers from Limitation to Proliferation', in the section entitled 'The Technicalities of Governing: Technologies, Government, Governmentality'.

A variety of literature is discussed in Chapter 2, 'Bio-politics, Normalcy and the Numerical Plotting of the Population', which allows for the subsequent analysis of dyslexia as a technology of power. Therein, I suggest that the period under investigation is one where relations of power had changed their emphasis. The activity of government became concerned with cultivating the population. The account presented by Michel Foucault in the final chapter of the *History of Sexuality Vol.1,* and in the lectures from the *Collège de France,* published as *Security, Territory, Population and the Birth of Politics,* are used as the point of departure to develop this argument in conjunction with research by Nikolas Rose (1999), Jacques Donzelot (1979, 1988, 1991), Ian Hacking (1982), Francois Ewald (1990, 1991), Mitchel Dean (1999), and Giles Deleuze and Felix Guattari (1987, 1988). These accounts provide material to develop an account of the process of capitalisation that I argue the population underwent during the nineteenth and early twentieth centuries. The population became a state's most valuable resource, and tactics of gov-ernment now utilised power to act upon both the body of individuals and the body of the population by proliferating skills, fostering abilities and directing their lives. Furthermore, these investigations allow me to sketch in greater detail the specific machineries of government, such as psychology, and specific technologies of power, such as normalcy, than Foucault gives in his initial account.

The norm is a significant technology of power for this project, as it comes to define how variation across and between populations shall be conceived. The norm becomes a technology of power that imbues particular moral significance onto individual bodies, by accrediting certain bodies as normal and others as deviating from the norm. It will be argued that the norm operated as a technology that imbued particular bodies with specific moral values depending on how they related to the norm.[5] I will explore how this particular technology of power allowed the population to be conceived of in a significantly different fashion and opened up the possibility of measuring deviations from what had come to be understood as normal. This, in turn, facilitated a variety of styles of government. The establishment of the norm led to the development of a variety of technologies of measurement—one of the most prominent and important of these being intelligence tests. The establishment of a variety of technologies of distinction allowed for a specific population to be acted upon by specialist techniques, made possible by the way these technologies of power altered the conception of the population. Dyslexia is positioned as a technology of power that was dependent upon the norm, as it identifies those who deviated negatively from accepted standards of literacy. Technologies of power perform specific operations, facilitating the flow of power onto particular sites, in particular directions and determining the substance of its flow. Technologies of power allow for the realisation of particular strategies of government. They operate in assemblage (Deleuze and Guattari, 1988: 398–9), plugging into one another allowing for more elaborate operations to be achieved. I have used the term 'machinery of government' to describe an assemblage of technologies of power that is being utilised by a strategy of government to achieve particular goals. Technologies, such as the norm, intelligence tests, ophthalmologic examinations and many more, at some point form part of the machinery of government that dyslexia is a component of.

In Chapter 3, 'Governing Readers from Limitation to Proliferation', I consider what strategies of government dyslexia facilities. I argue that the diagnostic category dyslexia is concerned with the proliferation of literacy. I try to describe the various factors that led to the enacting of this particular strategy of government. The chapter begins by explaining the way that the terms 'government' and 'governmentality' have been used in this book. I then argue that the invention of dyslexia as a technology of power should be understood as an event in the history of the government of reading. It is suggested that as governments became concerned with fostering the development of the population, the governing of reading shifted from a strategy of limitation to one of proliferation. Reading in these two different strategies refers to distinct activities, with different rationales and values attached. It is suggested that dyslexia as a technology of power is constituted to facilitate the strategy of the proliferation of literacy, or at least a certain level of literacy.

The strategies for governing reading are here contextualised as part of the development of bio-politics. The strategy of limitation is seen as an element of sovereign power and the strategy of proliferation as an element of a bio-political style of government. The historical investigations of Foucault (1979), Rose (1999) and Hacking (1982) are utilised to provide the context of my study, and their genealogical approach is also drawn upon to establish the methods I will be using to investigate the formation of dyslexia as a diagnostic category and as a technology of power.

This question is taken up in Chapter 4, 'Reading Difficulties Become a Medical Concern'. Here, an analysis of the formation of congenital word-blindness within the discipline of medicine is provided. The historical precedence of aphasia and various reading difficulties that are later cited by dyslexia researchers are explored. Kussmaul (1877) and Hinshelwood's (1895) work on acquired word-blindness is discussed. The silence in the literature between Schmidt (1600) (in Anderson and Meir-Hedde, 2001) and Kussmaul's (1877) papers provides the initial focus of the discussion. The formation of congenital word-blindness as a diagnostic category from research conducted into acquired word-blindness is then detailed. It is argued that acquired word-blindness makes medicine hospitable to the possibility of a congenital diagnosis concerned with reading difficulties. The primary analytical focus of Chapter 4 revolves around the question of how congenital reading difficulties became a legitimate concern for medical professionals. In this chapter it becomes apparent that if diagnostic categories are considered to be technologies of power, then they must perform particular operations, facilitating power to flow onto bodies in a specific way. The operation that congenital word-blindness is able to perform develops out of the operation that acquired word-blindness conducted.

In Chapter 5, 'The Technological Operation of Congenital Word-Blindness: Marking Some Differences as More Deserving than Others', the operation that congenital word-blindness performed as a technology of power is described in further detail. Focusing on the period after the initial research into congenital word-blindness when the diagnosis was ossifying, I describe how conflicting rationalities concerning the relative deservingness of the bodies accredited as congenitally word-blind resulted in slightly different versions of the diagnosis performing distinct operations. It is argued, therefore, that the operation that congenital word-blindness performs as a technology of power depends upon what strategy of government is enacting the technology, but also upon what rationalities of government were involved in its formation. Technologies of power therefore have many potential functions that are only realised when they are enacted and become technologies of government. The discussion is still very much dominated by ophthalmologists. Simultaneously, James Hinshelwood's status is developed by high praise provided in most of the research papers and conferences reports published during this time. The discussion of the 'deservingness' of these subjects is used to further outline how the diagnosis functioned. Consideration of how congenital word-blindness may operate as a technology of government is provided, and it is suggested that one of the key functions of the diagnosis is to operate as a mechanism of differentiation. The diagnosis served to distinguish between those whose difficulty with reading was seen to be an aspect of many other educational difficulties and those whose reading difficulty was considered to be a specific, isolated phenomena. The importance of this distinction is that those who are accredited with congenital word-blindness were able to be educated through specialised intervention. The hereditary and familial hypothesis gained currency across these papers, and this make the diagnosis as a technology of power more hospitable to forming rationalities of government that are directed to the biological stock of the population, such as eugenics and social hygienism.

In Chapter 6, 'Psychological Explanations for Congenital Word-Blindness', attention is given to describing various psychological accounts of reading difficulties. Particular attention is given to the Psychological Clinic at the University of Pennsylvania, and its associated journal. This institution and journal were both concerned with fostering direct links with schools. Many articles concerned with reading were thus published in the journal. This chapter thus describes how psychology began to develop a jurisdiction over the diagnosis as ophthalmology's influence waned. It suggested that psychology was successful in developing a jurisdiction, as institutions like the Psychological Clinic at the University of Pennsylvania were directly concerned with establishing links with schools and educational authorities. Their concern with establishing conduits through which their practices and technologies could disperse, and the particular focus on establishing links with schools, illustrates that elements within the discipline of psychology were directly concerned with making the school an increasingly hospitable site for psychological technologies and practices. Over time, this would position the characteristics that were being diagnosed as congenital word-blindness increasingly under the auspice of the discipline of psychology.

Chapter 7 is entitled 'The Problem of Producing Literate Subjects: Education and Specific Reading Difficulties'. This chapter describes the work of a variety of authors whose writings on reading in educational journals were one factor in making the school an increasingly hospitable site for a diagnosis such as congenital word-blindness. The discussion covers numerous areas: first, the processes by which children learn to read; second, the importance of pupils acquiring the ability to read to, in turn, develop a more advanced understanding of various subjects; third, the development of a concern that some pupils have a pronounced difficulty with reading; fourth, techniques for improving overall reading rates of a class and individuals accredited as having a difficulty; fifth, tests used to examine reading ability; sixth, the perceived social–cultural benefits of reading; and, seventh, the emergence of specific techniques for educating children accredited with congenital word-blindness. The purpose of these discussions is to provide a broader context of the attitudes that were emerging at the turn of the twentieth century regarding the skill of reading. It is hoped that this context will complement the analysis in previous chapters regarding the emergence of particular strategies of government and the importance that a literate population had for these strategies. The paramount importance of reading to so many facets of education is established, and further evidence is gathered for the contention that literate subjects were becoming ever more necessary to the emerging machineries of government as the twentieth century progressed. Particular attention is paid to the writings of Clara Schmitt, as she published the first article on congenital word-blindness in a teaching journal. This article is also the first time a considered and detailed approach to educating those accredited as having congenital word-blindness is developed, and it advocates improving those diagnosed with congenital word-blindness' literacy through the deployment of specifically described techniques. Her article on the test of mental ability is thus analysed in some depth. This is of particular relevance as these concerns are directly about reading. The majority of the other articles discussed have been culled from the *Elementary School*

Journal, where Schmitt published the aforementioned paper. I describe how a concern with reading developed within this journal, illustrating how it became possible to speak of congenital word-blindness within this particular professional grouping. The preceding chapters have been concerned with describing the necessary conditions for congenital word-blindness to be fashioned within the clinical disciplines of medicine, ophthalmology and psychology. The discussion now moves, for a time, away from mapping the conditions of possibility of diagnostic formation and analysing the diagnosis as a technology of power towards studying the process of its veridiction in a different field: schools. This allows for an understanding of how the diagnosis became a widely deployed technology in the pursuit of cultivating a literate population.

Chapter 8 concludes the book. I provide a summary of the formation of the diagnosis and its operation as a technology of power. I consider the invention of the diagnosis as an event in the history of reading. The contribution that my analysis provides to the analysis of power (described in Chapter 2) is outlined, and the genealogical study of impairment categories are positioned as necessary to our understanding of how particular human characteristics become problematic at different points in history.

Over the course of the chapters that follow I hope to make evident that separate, but related, events of the problematisation of a difficulty with reading and the invention of the diagnosis of 'dyslexia' are a response to two key shifts: first, a shift in the style of government—a shift towards treating bodies as a capitalised resource; and, second, a shift in the style of labour that these bodies are called on to perform, as the frequency of labour related to linguistic capacities increases.

It is hoped that mapping this genealogy will help to furnish a more nuanced understanding of how the specific problematisation of human characteristics occurred and how a particular diagnostic category—dyslexia—can be understood as illustrating a shift in the strategic priorities both of particular rationalities of government and also of the organisation of the economy. The genealogy that follows attempts to describe both the formation and deployment of a singular technology, which acts with many others in assemblage to mechanically produce the types of bodies most hospitable to the needs of the day.

I will now move on, in Chapter 2, to describe the work of various writers concerned with bio-politics. Describing the work of a variety of writers who understand the formation of particular technologies of power, or what I have called machineries of government, will be related to the shift in the style of power relations that bio-politics describe. I will begin by describing Foucault's (1979) description of this process before offering a discussion of various writers who have attempted to elaborate this argument through historical investigations. This discussion of bio-politics is provided so that the conditions of formation for the technology of power that I am concerned with—dyslexia—can be described. It is also necessary to provide this discussion to allow me to describe how dyslexia operated as a technology of power.

2
Bio-politics, Normalcy and the Numerical Plotting of the Population

In this chapter I will draw upon Foucault's work on the shift from sovereign power to bio-power. The exposition of this process draws upon historical and theoretical studies that have further elaborated Foucault's work concerning this transition. Through describing the changes in style, techniques and practices of government that took place during this period, I will outline the conditions that made the constitution of dyslexia as a diagnostic category possible. In this discussion I place particular importance on the invention and deployment of 'normality'; related developments in insurance and accounting; the emergence of disability as an administrative category; and changes in the perception of intelligence that occurred around the institutionalisation of psychology. This historical background serves to describe the invention and deployment of technologies of power, and particular shifts in the style of government that I consider to have constituted the material conditions that made dyslexia a possible, and subsequently widely deployed, diagnosis. In providing this context I am attempting to describe some of the conditions of possibility that allow the diagnostic category of dyslexia to be formed, to ossify and to be taken up by many different institutions, allowing me to describe and analyse, in the chapters that follow, the specific changes in practices of government and minute shifts in the operation of technologies of powers.

From Sovereign Power to Bio-power

Since its introduction in *History of Sexuality Vol.1 The Will To Knowledge* Foucault's concept of bio-power has functioned as a repeated point of departure for those seeking to develop academic collieries to new historical, political and philosophical perspectives on the body, government and the formation of numerous human sciences (Ewald, 1990; Rose, 1985, 1999). We find further elaboration on Foucault's conception of bio-politics and bio-power[1] in the series of lectures he gave at the Collège de France published as 'Security, Territory, Population' and 'The Birth of Biopolitics'. Bio-politics has proven to be a key concept for this project, as it describes a shift to a style of government that I am suggesting constituted the conditions that made dyslexia a possible diagnosis. It will thus be given extensive treatment in this chapter.

The *Will To Knowledge*, Foucault's first volume of the *History of Sexuality*, sees Foucault eschewing many of his previous theoretical developments regarding the analysis of power (Foucault, 1979: 135–59). *Discipline and Punish* carries the subtitle 'The Birth of the Prison', but the prison in question is not one with stone walls and bar-covered doors, but is instead the 'modern soul', the affect and instrument of the 'psy' sciences. The practices, technologies and academic disciplines that actively fashioned this soul are described. The axial point in this description is a shift in the style of punishment, a shift towards corrective institutions. The work provided a description of panoptic power relations, understanding power as disciplinary (Foucault, 1977: 195–228). *The Will to Knowledge* provided a new nexus around which an analysis of power could be developed—sexuality and confession, where the productive character of relations of power to incite discourse is described (Foucault, 1979: 17–35). Bio-power is a development of Foucault's analysis of disciplinary powers, reanimated with a productive character that considers the more complex, far-reaching and sometimes less visible operations that relations of power perform on the body (Foucault, 1979: 139–45).

Sexuality may not seem like the obvious target for an analysis of power in society. However, Foucault develops a unique approach to the political analysis of the individual body (Foucault, 1979: 139) and the body of the population (Foucault, 1979: 139–45), recognising that repression was a notion utilised by both individuals and the population to understand themselves. Foucault's analysis thus critiques both the Freudian theory of individual (sexual) repression and the Marxist theory of class oppression by substituting the 'repressive hypothesis' that our sexual life and our 'species being' (Marx, 1974) are repressed, with an analysis of power that emphasises its productive character. Power does not censor, veil, abstract or exclude. Instead, it produces reality; it produces domains of objects and regimes of truth (Butler, 2002: 13; Foucault, 1977: 194; Revel, 2008: 38). This theory of power recognises how our understanding of our body, objects and the institutions that govern us are constituted by relations of power that intertwine with relations of knowledge (Rose and Miller, 1992: 175). Discursive and non-discursive formations (Foucault, 1989a: 34–43) are run through by power relations that demarcate the limits of what can and cannot be considered to be a truthful statement (Foucault, 1979: 101–2). Foucault's research is thus best understood as a political history of truth (Foucault, 1979: 80) that challenges what allows truths to be spoken, to inform professional decisions and to govern the conduct of conduct (Foucault, 2000d: 220–1; Gordon, 1991: 2). Technologies of government delimit and manage the spaces in which we exist (Miller and Rose, 1990: 8), encouraging the proliferation of certain attributes (Foucault, 1979: 139), rather than estranging us from our 'species being' or natural 'psychological nature'.

Practices of government, according to Foucault's narrative, became, in the nineteenth century, peculiarly interested in the sexual practices of individuals, and, for the first time, the population was identified as a problem to be studied and as something to be governed (Foucault, 1979: 138–43, 2003: 253–63; Hacking, 1982: 281; Rose and Miller, 1992: 174). The population was now considered to be a resource, a phenomenon that could be utilised, altered and developed, to best serve the economic interests of the state. It thus became necessary for government to become concerned with the manner by which the population reproduces itself. For Foucault

> At the heart of this economic and political of population was sex: it was necessary to analyze the birth rate, the age of marriage, the legitimate births, the precocity and frequency of sexual relations, the ways of making them fertile or sterile, the effects of unmarried life or the prohibitions, the impact of contraceptive practises—of those notorious 'deadly secrets' which demographers on the eve of the Revolution knew were already familiar to the inhabitants of the countryside. (1979: 26)

The nineteenth century was characterised for Foucault by a shift in the way that power was exercised by government. According to Foucault, government previously primarily exercised sovereign power, characterised for him by the illustration that we find at the front of Hobbes's *Leviathan*. In this illustration the King's body is literately constituted by his people: they serve the King in the same way the hand of the King serves the King (Foucault, 1980: 121). This type of power was thus characterised by the King's sovereignty over the population and 'one of the characteristic privileges of sovereign power was the right to decide life and death' (Foucault, 1979: 135). The life of individual members of the population belonged to the King, so it was his right to decide whether individuals were to live or die. When Foucault's analysis turns towards the nineteenth century he suggests that a new strategy of government emerges, where power is exercised in a radically different fashion. He characterises this as 'bio-power' (Foucault, 1979: 138–43, 2003: 253–63). Bio-power contra sovereign power was characterised by the power over life contra the right of death (Foucault, 1979: 139). Relations of bio-power foster behaviours or attributes in the population.

Bio-power operates simultaneously at two different levels: at the level of the body of the individual, and at the level of the body of the population (Foucault, 2003: 253–63). The state, when exercising sovereign power, saw the body of the individual and the body of the population as nuisances that needed to be repressed so that the activity of government could continue unabated. Strategies of government that articulated relations of bio-power treated the body of the population and the body of the individual as a resource that, through careful intervention, could be maximised (Foucault, 1979: 138–143, 2003: 253–63). A bio-politics of the population conceives of the body as a resource, as capital. The manner by which educational institutions exercise power over the students is exemplary of how bio-power operates upon a population (Hunter, 1994). Students are organised into classes often based on their age or, in some cases, their accredited cognitive abilities (Jones and Williamson, 1979: 73). They are taught a curriculum that is framed by the political and moral judgements of educational policy makers (Hunter, 1988; Viswanathan, 1989), and, most importantly, it is assumed that most students will be, or can become, 'normal'. In Foucault's analysis the other pole that power operated through in this period was an anatamo-politics of the human body. Many of the technologies associated with this strategy of power used the matrix of the norm (Ewald, 1990: 141; Foucault, 1979: 139; Hacking, 1982: 279). The theme of normality and the reorganisation of life that takes place around this concept will be elaborated later in the chapter, and the articulation of relations of power by school and other educational institutions is discussed in Chapter 3.

Rabinow and Rose (2006), recognising the imprecision in Foucault's usage of the term, provide some clarification on the differences between bio-power and bio-politics—a distinction also affirmed by Lazzarato (2002):

> [W]hilst Foucault is imprecise in his use of the terms, it might be helpful to suggest that, within the field of biopower, we can understand

'biopolitcs' as the specific strategies and contestations over problematizations of collective human vitality, morbidity and morality. Over
the forms of knowledge, regimes of authority, and practices of intervention that are desirable, legitimate and efficacious. (Rabinow and
Rose, 2006: 198)

I shall distinguish between bio-power and bio-politics as follows. Bio-
power describes relations of power that are articulated upon the body
of the population with the intention of fostering particular attributes,
proliferating certain actions and managing risk (Rose, 1991: 677). Bio-
politics shall be used to describe a particular style of government[2] that
the articulation of many relations of bio-power in assemblage allowed
for the population to be cultivated as a resource—a style of government
where the population had been capitalised.

Elaborating the Bio-political Thesis

In *Homo Sacer* Giorgio Agamben argued 'The Foucauldian thesis will
then have to be corrected or, at least, completed' (1995: 9). Here, he
is referring to bio-politics that, for Agamben, is key to understanding
modern law and politics. Unlike many researchers deeply influenced
by Foucault's research on bio-power, Agamben, while recognising its
significance, is somewhat distrustful of Foucault's claim that the new
tactics of government associated with bio-power emerged in the nineteenth century. Agamben writes 'that Western politics is a Bio-politics
from the very beginning' (Agamben, 1995: 181). He argues further
that

> ...if in modernity life is more and more clearly placed at the centre of
> State politics (which now becomes, in Foucault's terms, Bio-politics),
> if in our age all citizens can be said, in a specific but extremely real
> sense, to appear virtually as *hominess sacri*, this is possible only
> because the relation of the ban has constituted the essential struc-
> ture of sovereign power from the beginning. (1995: 111)

A concern with the life of the population for Agamben has always characterised politics. I would argue that Agamben here is ignoring important empirical studies conducted in the wake of Foucault, which suggest
that the population was constituted in the early nineteenth century
(Ewald, 1990; Hacking, 1982, 1990, 1991).

Agamben contra Foucault argues that politics has always been concerned with life and its primary concern has been excluding individuals from being considered as citizens. The ban, the state of exception, outside or inside, exclusion or inclusion is, for Agamben, the original political relation (Agamben, 1995: 181). Power over life has always been implicit in any theory or practice of sovereignty. Bio-politics in Agamben's work separates populations by making some people less than human. While I agree that classification has been a central role of many of the technologies of power invented since the nineteenth century, and should, therefore, be central to any researcher concerned with bio-politics, I am concerned about drawing a line between ancient strategies of government and modern technologies of government. Agamben's analysis excludes this important historical and analytical distinction.

Foucault's research has typically been concerned with the manner in which power is exerted over life by an array of institutions and disciplines. The body, in Foucault's analysis, is reconstituted as a site affected by the government of the population (1979: 140–3 (bio-politics)) and political programmes concerned with individuals (1979: 139 (antamopolitics)). By arguing, as Agamben does, that politics has always been bio-political, the concept's ability to analyse the distinct technological shifts in strategies and practices of government during the nineteenth century (Castels, 1991; Defert, 1991; Donzelot, 1979, 1988, 1991; Ewald, 1990; Hacking, 1982, 1990, 1991; Miller, 1992; Rose, 1985, 1999) is neutered. Foucault's analysis diffuses the activity of government across society onto a wide range of institutions, whereas Agamben re-centres analysis upon the machinery of the state. Given that I am arguing that it is the technological innovations that occurred during the late nineteenth and early twentieth centuries that formed the conditions of possibility for dyslexia to be invented, the bio-politics I am operationalising are Foucauldian and not Agambenian.

In his study of the psychological complex (1985) Nikolas Rose asks the question 'In what ways, and with what consequences, did it become possible to think psychologically about the variations of capacities and attributes amongst individuals?' (Rose, 1985: 10) For Rose, this period is of interest because during it psychology leaves a speculative philosophical realm and attempts to imitate the natural sciences. Psychology in this period made use of many technologies of power that were being developed to plot the individual and the population numerically. Ian Hacking (1982, 1990, 1991) and Theodore M. Porter (1986) identified the period of 1850–1900 as the avalanche of printed numbers—a period where statistical technologies not only emerged as legitimate technologies for measuring the population, but also changed how we think about the population. This population and the individual could now be plotted numerically, and a new taxonomy was invented in response to this. For Hacking, this period marks the replacement of the laws of nature with statistics, probability and the norm (Hacking, 1990: 1). A similar analysis is presented by Rose, who states:

> This transformation can be partially understood in terms of the operation of the discourse of statistics. Statistics, the science of the state, had been initially conceived as the means to be deployed by statesmen in the determination of appropriate forms of legislation. (1985: 42–3)

Hacking (1990) argues that it was at this point that the population became governable in the way we understand it today. This numerical plotting of the population allowed it to be conceived of in the same fashion as another phenomenon that was described and governed numerically, namely capital. Like capital, the population became a resource; a resource that needed to be carefully managed to yield its greatest potential (Foucault, 1977: 141). Tactics of government changed as the population was refigured, in light of this numerical plotting, as a resource. As a result of this refiguring of the population, an array of new technologies concerned with acting upon the body of the population and cultivating it were invented. The way populations (both the population of the state and the populations of smaller institutions, such as the school, the company and the workhouse) are governed depends upon the technologies available to articulate relations of power onto and through the population. The invention of the population as an object of knowledge therefore accorded the state and various other institutions with the desire to know more and more about their population, as increased knowledge only augmented the potentials visible in these bodies (Rose and Miller, 1992: 174). Individual bodies and the body of the population were refigured as capital with many different potentialities, abilities and attributes; some were to be carefully managed and limited, while others were to be fostered and developed (Foucault, 1977: 141). The capitalisation of flesh made the body the site of potential activities of government. As relations of power circulated on and through it, more capillaries of resistance were opened up. It therefore became a site of increasing risk (Castels, 1991;

O'Malley, 2000). The question of what it means to govern shifted as a new problematic of government formed, where both the dangers and potentialities that were conceived as being presented in a population were augmenting:

> …the problem of population separated the question of its government from issues of trade, taxation production and the creation and circulation of wealth, it simultaneously freed these elements for their independent elaboration, for them to become the object of a specific discourse now termed in the nineteenth century, political economy. (Rose, 1985: 43)

The problems with which a state could legitimately consider to be under their jurisdiction therefore increased. The structure of the labour market was transformed; the type of labour that individuals undertook had changed. This shift towards thinking about individuals and populations as governable objects had been coupled with a dramatic transformation in the economic conditions of society. This shift was marked by an increased move to what Peter Drucker (1969) has called the knowledge economy and an increase in what Lazzarato (1996) has dubbed 'cognitive labour'. Skills, including literacy, now needed to be proliferated throughout the body of the population, as the individual and population were now conceived as a resource to be cultivated (Foucault, 1977: 141). Foucault dubbed this change in strategic thinking about the population the formation of a bio-politics of the population (Foucault, 1979: 140–3), while the change in thinking about the individual was dubbed to be the invention of an anatamo-politics of the individual (Foucault, 1979: 139):

> [Bi]o-power was without question an indispensable element in the development of capitalism; the latter would not have been possible without the machinery of production and the adjustment of the phenomena of population to economic processes. But this was not all it required; it also needed the growth of both these factors, their reinforcement as well as their availability and docility it had to have methods of power capable of optimising forces, aptitudes, and life in general without at the same time making them more difficult to govern. (Foucault, 1979: 140–1)

The process by which the articulation of bio-power, related to the development of capitalism, was making it possible for the population to be optimised or capitalised in the same way as other resources was described by Foucault as:

> The adjustment of the accumulation of men to that of capital, the joining of the growth of human groups to the expansion of productive forces and the differential allocations of profit, were made possible in part by the exercise of bio-power in its many forms and modes of application. The investment of the body, its valorisation, and the distributive management of its forces were at the time indispensable. (1977: 141)

The emergence of bio-political technologies of government made the individual an object of 'governmental' knowledge. The production of this new form of power allowed government to operate in ways that would have previously been inaccessible to the state. The body of the population and the body of the individual became objects accessible to the activity of government:

> ... the development of the great instruments of the state, as *institutions* of power ensured the maintenance of production relations, the power, ensured the maintenance of production relations, the rudiments of anatomo- and bio-politics, created in the eighteenth century as techniques of power present at every level of the social body and utilized by very diverse institutions (the family and the army, schools and the police, individual medicine and the administration of collective bodies), operated in the sphere of economic processes, their development and the forces working to sustain them. They also acted as factors of segregation and social hierarchization, exerting their influence on the respective forces of both these movements, guaranteeing relations of domination and effects of hegemony. (Foucault, 1977: 141)

The body became a malleable, adjustable, workable project once the 'body' of the population and the 'body' of the individual had been established as knowable, measurable and analysable objects of knowledge. The activity of government was no longer just under the jurisdiction of the state, but diffused throughout society (Deleuze and Guattari, 1988: 224). The government of the 'body' and 'soul' became the reasonability of numerous sectors of society—the family (Donzelot, 1979); the army (Foucault, 1979: 141); schools (Hunter, 1998, 1994; Jones and Williamson, 1979); medical practitioners (Foucault 1989b; Rose, 1985, 1999); the police (Pasquino, 1978); and numerous other groups.

The practices of government were now concerned with the harnessing of the productivity of individuals, and the minimising of 'risk' and 'moral degeneracy' (Jones and Williamson, 1979). A strategy of government concerned with the manipulation of the body with the intent of increasing economic productivity required the production of a certain type of body and a certain type of soul (Rose, 1999). This had been achieved through

> the proliferation of political technologies that invested the body, health, modes of subsistence and lodging—the entire space of existence in European countries from the eighteenth century onward. All the techniques that found their unifying pole in the limiting, repressive sense we give the term today, but according to a much boarder meaning that encompassed all the methods for developing the quality of the population and the strength of the nation. (Donzelot, 1979: 6)

This shift in tactics and techniques of government, and economic conditions, began to centre around a new mechanism: the norm (Davis, 1995; Ewald, 1990). It was a device that allowed for the cultivation of attributes in a population to be measured, acted upon and the success of the act to be judged. The normal body created a double problematic: normality was something to be exceeded if one was to be successful, but failure to attain the standards set by the norm marked bodies as unfit for purpose. This strategy of bio-political government required precise controls of the individual body to develop its complex economic, social and political systems.

The Reorganisation of Life: The Invention of *L'Homme Moyen*

> One can tell the story of biopolitics as the transition from the counting of hearths to the counting of bodies. The subversive effect of this transition was to create new categories into which people had to fall, and so to create and to render rigid new conceptualisations of the human being. (Hacking, 1982: 281)

We have not always been normal or abnormal; once, we were grotesque (Garland-Thomson, 1997: 56–63). The emergence of normality in the early nineteenth century enacted a new regime of truth around bodies, a regime that described bodies in numerical terms and marked them as inferior if they deviated from it (Davis, 1995; Ewald, 1990; Hacking, 1982, 1990, 1991). The declaring of a deviation as negative was informed by political, moral and economic judgements.

An early consideration of normality was provided by the French historian of science George Canguilhem in *The Normal and the Pathological* (1989). Here, Canguilhem asserts that 'our image of the world is always a display of values as well' (Canguilhem, 1989: 179). This classic of the history of science approaches the 'sciences of life' in a Nietzschean fashion so as to question the political, moral and subjective values that are present in our images of normality (Canguilhem, 1989: 45; Foucault, 2000: 465–77). Canguilhem underlines how a contemporary understanding of the human condition would be impossible without the technologically, politically, economically and statistically determined concepts of normality and pathology. It is necessary to follow Canguilhem in studying the social, political, technological and moral factors that have constructed particular abnormalities, and thus excluded them from the ever-shrinking space of 'normality'.

Canguilhem studies the invention of the concepts of the normal and pathological to produce a critique of these concepts (Canguilhem, 1989: 289). Although Canguilhem studied these concepts in terms of medicine and biology, the norms constituted in these disciplines are often translated in juridical norms, making this study relevant to the analysis of bio-power. There is a twofold reason for this research's relevance to this study as I am concerned with the formation of a diagnosis in medical discourse that relies upon the existence of certain norms. Canguilhem alerts us to how the development of statistics allows for the conception of 'norms'[3]: '[w]ithout doubt there is one way to consider the pathological and normal and that is by defining normal and abnormal in terms of relative statistical frequency' (Canguilhem, 1989: 137). Statistics transferred the norm from being the concern of medicine and biology to being a technology of power articulated in numerous fields.

Pathology is constituted as a deviation from the normal state. Prior knowledge of the normal state is required before something can be judged to be pathological, 'but conversely the scientific study of pathological cases becomes an indispensable phase in the overall search for the laws of the normal state' (Canguilhem, 1989: 51). The normal and the pathological thus operate in a feedback loop, with more pathologies being developed as a greater number of standards are made visible that the body is supposed to adhere to.

Canguilhem deals with a key problem brought about by the conflation of the normal and the average:

> On the whole the physiologists who reviews its basic concepts is well
> aware that for him norm and average are two inseparable concepts.
> But average seems to him to be directly capable of objective defini-
> tion so he tires to join the norm to it. (1989: 156)

This conflation is problematic as the two concepts are not as similar
as they first seem. The problem resonates beyond the confines of the
disciplines where norms are formed, as scientific norms are translated
into juridical norms (Canguilhem, 1992: 248). This becomes increasingly problematic as the norm is imbued with moral values (Davis,
1995; Ewald, 1990). Canguilhem's project ultimately draws our attention to the relativity of norms depending on our environment; what is
normal to one organism in one setting will not be normal to another
in a different environment (Canguilhem, 1989: 239–40). The types of
activities that humans engage in alter their norms, in turn changing
how humans relate to their environment:

> Each of us fixes his norms by choosing his models of exercise. The
> norm of a long-distance runner is not that of a sprinter. Each of us
> changes his norms according to his age and former norms. The norm
> of the former sprinter is not that of a champion...This recognition of
> the individual and chronological relativity of norms is not scepticism
> before multiplicity but tolerance of variety. (Canguilhem, 1989: 284)

Canguilhem's rethinking of the normal and the pathological in biology and medicine undermines the principles that underlie eugenic and
social hygienic strategies of government, as both eugenicism and social
hygienism are rationalities of government that rely not only upon various articulations of the technology of the norm, but a norm that has
been imbued with an array of moral forces (Rose, 1984: 363–99). The
expression of the norm in these rationales of government was archaic,
even in its first articulations. The normal, when deployed by strategies of government that utilise an anatamo-politics of the human
body or a bio-politics of the population, develops a meaning beyond its
etymology as:

> *norma*, etymologically means a T-square, normal is that which bends
> neither to the right nor left, hence that remains in a happy medium;

from which two meanings are derived 1) normal is that which is such that it ought to be; 2) normal, in the most usual sense of the word, is that which is met with in the majority of cases of a determined kind, or that which constitutes either the average or standard of a measurable characteristic. (Canguilhem, 1989: 125)

Canguilhem's influence was significant across post-1945 French thought, but the influence was particularly strong upon Foucault (1998c: 465–77, 2001: 255–6) and his circle. Francois Ewald, a student and collaborator of Foucault's, places the normal at the centre of his elaboration of Foucault's work on bio-politics. The influence of Canguilhem here is evident (Ewald, 1990: 139). Ewald draws attention not only to the movement of norms across various bureaucratic and scientific fields, but also to its expansion in the French language. As an augmentation of the number fields where the norm is articulated increases

> [t]he vocabulary associated with the term expands as well: in French, normal is no longer the only way to derive from *norme*. It is joined by *normalité* (1834) *normatif* (1868), and *normalisation* (1920). This remarkable extension of the norm's domain will affect a wide variety of fields concerned with economics and technology. It will also have a major influence on the moral, juridical, and political sciences...(Ewald, 1990: 140)

The norm is a technology through which power is articulated in a variety of different disciplines, by various institutions and onto different types of bodies. When deployed in these different sites the norm operates in assemblage with a large variety of technologies of power. The centrality of the norm in the development of a bio-politics of the population out of the technologies associated with an anatamo-politics of the individual is described by Ewald:

> The norm is the principle that allows discipline to develop from a simple set of constraints into a mechanism; it serves as the matrix that transforms the negative restraints of the juridical into the more positive controls of normalization and helps to produce the generalization of discipline. (1990: 141)

Ewald (1990) argues that the norm allowed disciplinary powers to be generalised across the entire population. As power flowed through the matrix that the norm provided, the character of these relations of power alerted and became increasingly productive. Disciplinary techniques of power could be generalised onto the population through the moralised standards that the norm offered. This is because the norm allowed for comparisons to be made between bodies, judging them against this technology of measurement. The norm is here being positioned as the technology that allows for power to develop an increasingly productive character concerned not with restricting bodies but with re-producing them. While I am wary of seeing disciplinary power as repressive, as Ewald (1990) seems to imply, I do agree that it was in assemblage with this particular technology of power that a variety of mechanisms for governing the population were able to be generalised and the productivity of relations became common knowledge to those concerned with government.

Power could now focus both on the individual body and the body of the population. Both of these bodies were capitalised, and the bifocal character was partly generated by the mechanism of the norm. Ewald describes how Quetelet's average man operated as an instrument by which a population could be evaluated by reference to itself (the importance of Quetelet's average man, or *l'homme moyen*, in reordering the population is also described by Davis (1995), Garland Thomson (1997) and Hacking (1990)). *L'homme moyen* performed a function synonymous with the function that the norm performed in medicine and biology, identifying deviations from its measure as being pathological. One of the ways that the norm is operationalised in a bio-politics of the population is through Quetelet's average man:

> With his theory of the average man, Quetelet proposes a means of specifying individuals with reference to their position within a group, rather than playing close attention to their essence, their nature, or their ideal state of being. The theory of the average man, their nature, or their idea state of being. The theory of the average man, then, is an instrument that makes it possible to understand a population with respect only to itself, and without recourse to some external defining factor. (Ewald, 1990: 146)

A population could be measured against itself without the need for an external factor, without the need for an ideal. It is this instrument that makes population autonomous. Through this, the population became a discernable object of knowledge. It became something that could be acted upon, and strategies of government responded by reformulating how they saw the population as a resource. The population became capital (Foucault, 1977: 141).

The reorganisation of life around the poles of normality and abnormality, and the concurrent capitalisation of the population, should, in my opinion, be considered as an important event for historians of disablement as industrialisation. Many pre-existing impairment categories were codified in this period, and impairment categories were formulated in response to this reorganisation. Within disability studies one of the most vocal critics of 'normalcy' has been Lennard Davis. His study, 'Enforcing Normalcy', describes how disability operates in relation to the concept of the norm:

> The term 'disability', as it is commonly and professionally used, is an absolute category without a level or threshold. One is either disabled or not. One cannot be a little disabled more than one be a little pregnant [...] A concept with such a univalent stronghold on meaning must contain within it a dark side of power, control, and fear. (1995: 1)

This absolute concept operates by evoking the diagram of the norm and asserting that those marked as disabled cannot be situated within the boundaries of 'normality'. Disability, for Davis, is a social process that involves everyone, as we are all embodied beings. 'Just as the conceptualization of race, class and gender shapes the lives of those who are not black, poor or female the concept of disability regulates the body of those who are "normal"' (Davis, 1995: 1). From the start of his book on deafness, Davis asserts that this is a book about normal bodies and abnormal bodies. It is a history of how deafness has become considered to be an impairment, and how a deaf person is considered to have an abnormal body. This is a process of exclusion from 'normality'. The book is concerned with the invention of normalcy, and how this reconstituted individuals who do not fit within this regimented categories to being formulated as subjects of alterity.

Davis's book rests upon two axes or, rather, is directed by two problems. First: How is it that one comes to consider themselves and others as normal? Second: How is it that one can become considered as abnormal by themselves and/or others? Through Davis's analysis perhaps we can begin to understand the category of disability as a technology for governing difference, a technology that operates in assemblage with a variety of technologies specific to impairment categories. How are we to understand the operation of this assemblage of impairment categories and disability? 'To understand the disabled body, one must return to the concept of a norm, the normal body'. (Davis, 1995: 23).

Davis describes the process by which the construction of the normal body differentiates the disabled body. He also warns that this must not, however, be separated from a wider study of the evasiveness of norms in our culture: 'There is probably no area of contemporary life in which some idea of a norm, mean, or average has not been calculated' (Davis, 1995: 23). The norm is a technology of power that incites individuals to continually measure themselves against it. Our earnings, political choices, ethical choices, thoughts and consumption patterns are measured against *l'homme moyen*. Our sex drive, weight, height, cholesterol level, intelligence, etc., are conceptualised in relation to a narrow spectrum of normality. For instance, the statistical concepts of subnormality and above-average are embedded as qualitative moral values—we are to feel inferior about ourselves if one is subnormal and good about oneself if one is above average. The norm is thus not just something to be achieved but something to be exceeded. Medical provision relies upon the statistical average to understand our health. Educational institutions plot children's measured intelligence and attainment upon normal curves, dispense standardised tests that are dependent upon norms and classes are then segmented based upon these instruments. It should be recognised that this recently formulated framework imposes itself like a grid onto organic and non-organic matter declaring where life begins and where it ends. Life, as it will be argued later in the chapter, becomes synonymous with normalcy, and if one recedes under the diagrammed line of normality then one's ability to live life is called into question. A demarcation as less than normal is a diagnosis that may, of course, lead to technological, moral or social support, but commonly it will come hand in hand with a life-sentence of domination, where capillaries of resistance become clogged.

I have become increasingly convinced of the importance of Quetelet's concept of *l'homme moyen* after surveying literature concerned with the development of new scientific disciplines—individual psychology (Rose, 1985, 1999); technologies of government; statistics (Hacking, 1982, 1990, 1991); insurance (Defert, 1991; Ewald, 1990, 1991; Miller, 1992); the importance of the norm for the formation of institutions (such as the clinic (Foucault, 1989b), the prison (Foucault, 1977) and the school (Hunter, 1988, 1994))—and an array of new diagnostic categories (including the normal and abnormal (Cangiulhem, 1989; Davis, 1995; Ewald, 1990), madness (Foucault, 2006), the homosexual (Foucault, 1979) and disability (Garland-Thomson, 1997: 64–7)), which were invented during the late nineteenth and twentieth centuries. *L'homme moyen* synthesised *l'homme moyen physique* and *l'homme moyen morale*; both were remarkably important to the development of the social relations that made a diagnosis such as dyslexia technically possible and bureaucratically useful. Quetelet's average man was constructed as the morally and physically average human. It became central to the workings of capitalist societies providing an ontological foundation upon which disciplines are produced and government operated (Davis, 1995; Ewald, 1990; Foucault, 1977, 1979; Garland-Thomson, 1997; Hacking, 1982, 1990; Procacci, 1978; Rose, 1985, 1999). These various technical and bureaucratic changes altered how individuals and societies were conceived (Hacking, 1990: 4).

Although he does not explicitly draw attention to the political implications, Davis (1995) rightly recognises the societal implications of the introduction of *l'homme moyen*, as it provides a scientific justification formulated for the value of moderation and the middle class morality of *les classes moyens*. These moral values are attached to the technology of normality. Davis (1995) emphasises how these relations of power have resulted in the constitution of sciences that would justify the political positioning of the norm. Middle class ideology thus framed what was considered to be normal, and normality gave a scientific justification to the political and moral programs of *les classes moyens*. If we consult the work of Ewald (1990, 1991, 2002), Foucault (1979, 2003), Rose (1985, 1987, 2001, 2006) and histories of disability (Davis, 1995; Garland-Thomson, 1997; Stiker, 1997) it becomes evident how important the constitution of *l'homme moyen* was for the transformation of individuals previously seen as extraordinary or grotesque, or, conversely, where no difference was apparent, to become understood as normal or abnormal. This refiguring of life, with bodies now relating to a new set of diagrams (Deleuze, 1992: 22), normal and abnormal, meant that impairment categories were now to be plotted in relation to these concepts. Physical normalcy and moral normalcy became entwined; sexual, physical, cognitive and moral difference could now be codified as 'abnormal'; the rules of what it meant to be 'normal' were written through investigations into so-called abnormality. In his 1974–75 lecture course *Abnormal*, Foucault (2003), analyses a variety of such cases, including, amongst others, cannibalism; possessions; the masturbator; and 'Siamese twins'. Being accredited as abnormal only identified a physical or cognitive difference. It alluded to an abnormal individual being morally dubious because there was now an obligation to be normal (Davis, 1995: 29; Garland-Thomson, 1997: 32).

Across the nineteenth century the norm, or one of its derivatives, was articulated in an increasing array of sites (Ewald, 1990: 148;

Garland-Thomson, 1997: 42; Hacking, 1982: 282, 1990: 1). The norm was so successful in reordering the bodies of individuals and the population that it became difficult to imagine that the norm had not existed:

> To those who first worked on normalization, the concept appeared as a sort of universal ordering principle. All the institutions that make society possible, no matter how primitive, such as language, writing, money instruments of measurements, habits and customs, all suddenly seemed to derive, at least in retrospect, from practices of normalization. The normalizing process had accompanied humanity in every stage of its development. It served a primary social function by regularizing human conduct and by facilitating both technical progress and communication. No social object could escape normalization, and society would be inconceivable without it, for norms and standardization had always played an essential role in social development. (Ewald, 1990: 148)

It is hard to think of a social process where the norm was not deployed in some way as a technology of regulation. The success of the norm is made apparent when we consider that the concept, used in the modern sense, is not yet 200 years old (Davis, 1995; Hacking, 1990). Moreover, it is hard to imagine how the world was ordered prior to its existence. Through its articulation onto the body of the population and the body of the individual:

> Normalization forces each individual to imagine the ordering principle behind his activity not only with respect to some ideal of perfection that he might attain in isolation (such an ideal isolation has no meaning in a normative system), but with respect to a determined need that must be satisfied. Normalization is a means of organizing that solidarity which makes each individual the mirror and measure of his fellow. (Ewald, 1990: 151)

As has been described above, scientific, political and moral developments would not be possible without the invention and subsequent dominance of 'normalcy'. Rose (1979, 1985, 1987, 1996a, 1996b, 1999) eloquently and incisively draws our attention towards two divergent developments of the late nineteenth and early twentieth centuries— eugenic politics and the psychology of the individual, a further innovation that relies upon the technologies of normalcy. Rose describes how psychology in this period changed. It became less speculative, less philosophical, and it began to look toward the natural sciences for its models. The emergence of experimental individual psychology was thus made possible by technological changes in statistics—specifically the development of normal curves and intelligence tests. The logic upon which it was developed became mathematical rather than linguistic (Guattari and Alliez, 2010: 233). The technological shifts allowed psychological sciences to change, but economic changes and shifts in political desire encouraged and furthered this transformation. The psychological revolution was thus a result of the changing ways of governing the population, and then later a significant contributor to the possibility of government. The formation of the disciplinary character of individual psychology facilitated the operation of particular technologies of power associated with bio-politics, the development of a wide array of technologies of power associated with psychology that were dependent upon the norm and the ability to plot individuals numerically. How this impacted on the development of specific technologies of power toward producing the diagnosis of dyslexia is discussed in Chapter 7.

The argument is often made that statistics (Elden, 2006; Miller, 1992; Miller and Rose, 1990; Rose, 1991) have made it possible for the government to think of individuals and populations in numerical terms, thus allowing for the development of an array of technologies for measuring individuals and populations that, in turn, allowed for new strategies of government to be conceived. Ian Hacking (1982, 1990, 1991) has worked to describe the invention of statistical technologies and the resulting tactics of government that were made possible by the development of these specific technologies. Rose (1991) argues that since 'the avalanche of printed numbers' described by Hacking (1981) 'numbers' have become 'integral to the problematizations that shape what is to be governed, to the programmes that seek to give effect to government, and to the unrelenting evaluation of the performance of government that characterises modern political culture' (Rose, 1991: 675).

The emergence of the 'norm', in its modern English usage is dated by Davis (1995) between the years 1840 and 1860. Significantly, Hacking (1982) dubs a similar period, 1830–1848, the *avalanche of printed numbers*; a period during which there was a dramatic augmentation of statistical documents. Harold Westergaard (1932) describes a similar period in a comparable fashion that he dubs *the era of enthusiasm for statistical data collection*.

Statistics rendered the population understandable in numerical terms, referring to the statistical bureaus that were established across

Europe (Hacking, 1990: 34). Hacking states that 'The institutions brought a new kind of man into being the man whose essence was plotted by a thousand numbers' (Hacking, 1990: 34). The individual and the population were transformed by the ability to plot their various attributes numerically. Mechanisms of data collection became in themselves technologies for producing the individual and the population. However, statistics did more than map the attributes of individuals and populations in an avalanche of printed numbers (Hacking, 1982). They allowed for accidents to be transformed into risks, as chance was tamed:

> Statistics, in enabling the taming of chance, in turning a qualitative world into information and rendering it amenable to control, in establishing the classifications by which people come to think of themselves and their choices, appears to be bound with an apparatus of domination. (Rose, 1991: 677)

The numerical plotting of information about individuals and the population enabled the development of many precise technologies and strategies of government that would have been unthinkable before individuals and populations could be described numerically. Events and accidents could be studied and mathematically modelled, chance was no longer something to be feared, but something that could be studied and, ultimately, managed (Hacking, 1990). This taming of chance meant that accidents could be insured against, likely sites could be identified and methods could be developed for dealing with the risks they faced (Castels, 1991; Defert, 1991; Ewald, 1990, 1991; Miller, 1992). The number of relations of power that the state could articulate augmented drastically, as mathematical models allowed for the development of practices of government that were more complex than ever previously imagined (Bell, 1993; Burchell, 1991, 1996; Dillon, 1995; Elden, 2002; Hunter, 1998; Larner and Walters, 2004; O'Malley, 2000; Rose, 1993, 1999; Rose and Miller, 1992; Valverde, 1996).

The construction of 'normality' and a move to strategies of government directed by a numerical ontology are entwined with one another to the extent that each of these technologies made the world more amenable to the other. This is not to suggest that numerical thinking, or the concept of the norm, are intrinsically evil, or even bad (Foucault, 1997b: 343). Numbers have not engendered domination. As Rose claims, it is rather that in 'modern democratic discourse, numbers are thus not univocal tools of domination, but mobile and polyvocal resources' (Rose, 1991: 684). Like everything else they are dangerous rather then evil (Foucault, 1997b: 343). Understanding the population in mathematical terms will not inherently lead to the domination of the population. Instead, it opens as many capillaries of resistance as conduits for power to flow (Foucault, 1997c: 167; Lazzarato, 2002; Revel, 2008). Mathematical ways of conceptualising bodies are not inherently, morally and politically dubious. Instead, the strategies that have been deployed by the state and the human sciences have been formulated in relation to moral and political positions. The entwining of numerical strategies of government, *l'homme moyen* and particular political and moral judgements, has been hinted towards by Davis (1995), but not analysed. The strength of genealogical accounts and the accounts of those associated with governmentality is that they analyse how various discursive and non-discursive formations have interacted to produce other discourses and to frame objects. The strength of the genealogical method is in attention to minutia, and its concern with analysing rather then explaining (Foucault, 1998a).

The introduction of the concept of normality reordered and transformed how the population was thought and how it could be acted upon. This reordering produced new capillaries through which power could flow, and a series of other technologies were engineered that built upon these developments (statistics, intelligence tests, insurance). These technologies aimed to nurture the newly malleable population:

> The norm is equalizing; it makes each individual comparable to all others; it provides the standard of measurement. Essentially, we are all alike and, if not altogether interchangeable, at least similar, never different enough from one another to imagine ourselves as entirely apart from the rest. If the establishment of norms implies classification, this is primarily because the norms creates classes of equivalency. (Ewald, 1990: 154)

It has, therefore, been hard to separate these technologies of power from the study of the norm because the norm was deployed so purposefully. The norm is a technology of power that only operated in assemblage with other mechanisms. It often served as an amplifier, allowing power to flow deeper into the body of an individual or the population. As the norm became a measure more aspects of our lives were measured against classifications generated as differences that were not visible prior to the mathematical modelling of humans. Statistics, as a technology of government, therefore make visible and (more importantly) measurable the differences between a wide array of seemingly distinct groups.

Correlations can be formulated between particular social characteristics and behaviours or features of the population that are considered problematic. Government can thus become focused upon eliminating or at least minimising characteristics and behaviour viewed as problematic, and proliferating characteristics considered beneficial.

Ian Hacking's (1982, 1990, 1991) argument that the emergence of the science of the state through statistics engendered the possibility of new practices for governing the population is a well rehearsed and often repeated thesis. The rapid rise of bio-political techniques of government (ways of governing focused on regulating the body of the population, and attempting to maximise its productivity and minimise its risk), were made possible by the attempts to gather huge amounts of data about the population, which, in turn, came from a desire to develop a bio-political strategy of government. Hacking quotes Engels describing how the machinery of statistical measurement follows an individual throughout their life, recording information to be analysed and measured at every juncture:

> In order to obtain an accurate representation, statistical research accompanies the individual through his entire earthly existence. It takes account of his birth, his baptism, his vaccination, his schooling and the success thereof, his diligence, his leave of school, his subsequent education and development; and, once he becomes a man, his physique and his ability to bear arms. It also accompanies the subsequent steps of his walk through life; it takes not of his chosen occupation, where he sets up his household and his management of the same; if he saved from the abundance of his youth for his old age, if and when and at what age he marries and who he chooses as his wife—statistics looks after him when things go well for him and when they go awry. Should he suffer a shipwreck in his life, undergo material, moral or spiritual ruin, statistics takes note of the same. Statistics leaves a man only after his death and noted the causes that brought about his end. (Engels, 1862, quoted in Hacking, 1990: 34)

As the statistical plotting of every aspect of an individual's life became necessary to the operation of government, a variety of '[c]ategories had to be invented in which people could conveniently fall in order to be counted' (Hacking, 1990: 3). Segmenting a population into smaller populations now made sense, as their different characteristics could be plotted mathematically. Bio-politics therefore took on micro-political operations (Deleuze and Guattari, 1988: 211–13). Problematic aspects of particular populations could be managed, and attributes in individuals that were considered to be desirable could be fostered (Foucault, 1979: 138–43, 2003: 253–63). To some extent statistics actually constituted the body of the population, making it material in the sense that it could managed, acted upon and improved (Hacking, 1990: 6). All this was made possible by the ability to measure and record a group, comparing the results to see if the strategies of government had been successful.

In addition to the invention of a variety of technologies and mechanisms of data collection 'The very thought of being representative had to come into being' (Hacking, 1990: 6–7). This necessitated the development not only of vast machineries of government for counting people, because '[a]n entire style of scientific reasoning had to evolve' (Hacking, 1990: 6–7). The desire or 'professional lust for precision in measurement, were driven by familiar themes of manufacture, mining, trade, health, railways, war, empire. Similarly the idea of a norm became codified in these domains' (Hacking, 1990: 5). The non-discursive domain of the economy was thus interacting with statistical technologies, encouraging them to develop in particular directions. All the while the norm was becoming firmly attached to an increasing number of sites (Davis, 1995; Ewald, 1990; Garland-Thomson, 1997). A style of scientific reasoning and a strategy for governing the population was being constituted in relation to the economy. Economic thinking was being articulated into the practice of governing the population. It is not surprising therefore that the population came to be capitalised (Foucault, 1977: 141).

The capitalisation of the population led to the development of rationales of government concerned with assuring the continued profitability of this new resource. Giddens (1999: 3) describes a society that is preoccupied with the future that generates the notion of risk. This style of thought that was invented was based upon what Hacking calls '[t]he most decisive conceptual event of twentieth century physics has been the discovery that the word is not deterministic' (Hacking, 1990: 1). This discovery changed how the population could be governed. Ewald (1990: 142) describes how the practice of insurance emergences out of a formalisation of probability, as the combination of the taming of chance (Hacking, 1990) and the mathematical modelling (Ewald, 1990; Hacking, 1982, 1990) of the population provided the technical means by which the future could be governed. Technologies of insurance formalise the calculation of probability. The insurer 'produces risks by making them visible and comprehensible as such in situations where the individual would ordinarily see only the unpredictable hazards of his or her particular fate' (Ewald, 1990: 142). The cost of the unpredictable can now be managed through insurance policies.

So in allowing for the calculation of risk and the subsequent government of risk, the unpredictable character of life becomes more manageable. The diffusion of insurance and risk throughout society was one of the processes that augmented the capitalisation of the population. Risk here is the mechanism by which a certain kind of individual is assembled, and a particular type of population is formed. Manageable risk segmented the population, altering what problematics could to be governed as future events became an increased concern (Ewald, 1990: 146). The taming of chance and the creation of the norm reshaped bureaucratic thinking, necessitating the creation of an array of new technologies of government. As risk and insurance (Donzelot, 1991: 84) were proliferated through the machinery of government, the numerically-plotted individuals and population were increasingly governed by the calculative practices of accounting (Miller, 2001: 394).

The numerical plotting of the population and individuals made calculations possible which had previously been reserved for resources. The body was now subject to a new array of technologies of power—those associated with accounting. They provide an array of mechanisms through which individual achievements could be compared with financial norms and standards, the vocabulary of cost and costliness was articulated into the body of individuals and the population (Miller, 2001: 385). This individualised performance, by encouraging individuals to consider themselves as calculating selves, built upon the developments of statistics and the norm as 'individuals [were] rendered calculable and comparable' (Miller, 2001: 380). Government could translate 'diverse and complex processes into a single *financial figure*' (Miller, 2001: 381). As individuals were increasingly described as financial figures, it is not surprising that there was a rise in technologies of power concerned with improving their attributes.

Many of the technical innovations I have been describing provide the new laws that life is governed by:

> A new type of law came into being, analogous to the laws of nature, but pertaining to people. These new laws were expressed in terms of probability. They carried with them the connotations of normalcy and of deviations form the norm. The cardinal concept of the psychology of the Enlightenment had been, simply, human nature. By the end of the nineteenth century, it was being replaced by something different: normal people. (Hacking, 1990: 1)

The world was now inhabited not only by normal and abnormal people, but also by calculable people, as finance and risk were kneaded into the individual and population, further capitalising their flesh. This body diagrammed anew, plotted by a thousand numbers, took on an immaterial character as it became calculable beyond the immediate faculties of the five human senses. The diagnostic category dyslexia is a complex formulation that would be technically infeasible without these technologies contributing to the diagramming of the human through the vision of numbers rather then the eyes of man. These innovations changed the terrain of government, and a diagnosis that would mark a precise population as having a specific difficulty with reading was now a logical possibility. If literacy was to be proliferated throughout the population then both identifying bodies where standard methods of instruction were not successful and generating techniques to cultivate the necessary attributes became rationale. In this chapter I have described the invention of the rationale and technical means that make dyslexia a feasible diagnosis.

Conclusion

Liberal governmentalities are concerned with the production of 'productive docile bodies' and minimising risk (Dean, 1999: 176–97; Dillon, 1995). The development of statistical analysis in the early nineteenth century (Hacking, 1982) made possible the differentiation of groups that were unproductive or could cause 'risk' in the deployment of social welfare policies (Donzelot, 1991; Ewald, 1990, 1991). The government of the population has been made more effective by the analysis of groups 'in poverty', 'in poor health' or 'poorly educated', as well as identifying groups that are the inverse of this, i.e. 'well educated'. This segmentation of the population has been made possible by large-scale statistical analysis. The invention of statistics allowed for the fragmentation, segmentation and construction of groups in the population who were at 'risk' of being poorly educated and in poor health, and therefore facilitated the creation of categories of understanding. These would not exist without statistics and other mathematical ways of understanding society. Bodies could now be described in how far they deviated from norms. Indeed, as has been shown, the modern understanding of normality was invented during the 1820s. Bodies could be counted as part of segmented populations.

With the invention of the Binet-Simon test in the first decade of the twentieth century the cognitive capacities of individuals could be measured. The development across the proceeding decades of further psychological technologies concerned with measuring individual attributes allowed for further ways of classifying individuals to be developed. All of this allowed for the development of a style of strategies of government concerned with risk. Risk could now be calculated and insured against. As the nineteenth century progressed the activity of government increasingly relied upon mathematical foundations, and this augmented further in the first decades of the twentieth century. In response to these technological changes many technologies of power with a microscopic focus were able to be developed. Perhaps the art of government was undergoing a process of formalisation into a science. A scientific activity requires precise instruments capable of performing small and specialised operations. In the chapters that follow I shall investigate whether the diagnostic category of dyslexia was one such instrument.

3
Governing Readers from Limitation to Proliferation

In this chapter the concepts of government, strategy of government, governmentality and a variety of associated concepts shall be elaborated upon. The government of reading will then be analysed to describe how a shift in the strategy of governing literacy helped to constitute dyslexia's conditions of possibility. These concepts help to provide a theoretical framework, and illuminate the empirical context that makes it possible for me to conduct the precise genealogy of this diagnostic category, a technology of power—dyslexia. This book primarily studies the operations of technologies of power. I am not studying the formation of a governmentality, but rather how they relate to technologies of power. It is necessary to develop a more elaborate description of government and governmentality so that it is evident that my analysis of technologies and machineries of government refer back to a particular reading of the usage of the concepts of government and governmentality in the post-Foucauldian genealogical tradition.

The development of the printing press in the 1450s and the resulting ability to mass produce texts is briefly described, and it is suggested that this led to a change in how texts were related to, and, in turn, how reading was considered. I then use a small selection of secondary sources to suggest that prior to the development of bio-political styles of government reading was governed by a strategy of limitation. Reading was governed in this way because it was understood to be a particularly potent attribute; an attribute that was considered to be dangerous if widely distributed throughout the body of the population. As such, a strategy of limiting how many people had access to this attribute was deployed. Material culled from the Hansard transcriptions of parliamentary debates are then used to illustrate how a different strategy to govern reading was established. This strategy was initially disciplinary in its character and was concerned with producing docile bodies. However, it eventually became concerned with proliferating reading skills throughout the body of the population. I then describe the operation of two of the technologies' proliferation—the school and English literature—utilising a variety of studies and some primary sources to establish how these operated.

The Technicalities of Governing: Technologies, Government, Governmentality

Between the first and second volumes of the *History of Sexuality*, Michel Foucault gave a series of lectures around the topic of governmentality. These were the final lectures of 'Society Must be Defended' (2003) and the course, 'Security, Territory, Population' (2007). These themes were then further developed in the course on the *Birth of Biopolitics*. My usage of the concept of government here draws upon these lectures, but employs a variety of other research to correct some of its potential deficiencies. First, it must be stated that the study of government enacted in this book is not concerned only, or primarily, with the state as a centre of the operation of power (Deleuze and Guattari, 1988: 224). Instead, it is defined in the widest possible sense as the 'conduct of conduct', an activity that is diffused throughout society (Dean, 1999; Foucault, 2000d: 220–1, Gordon, 1991: 2). Furthermore, it must be clarified that the approach being integrated is formed by the diverse array of writers that Mitchell Dean (1999) refers to as working with the 'governmentality paradigm'.[1] These studies pioneered new ways of researching the practices, technologies and rationalities of government. They also developed their concepts of government from Foucault's re-conceptualisation of power that I described in Chapter 2.

In light of this re-conceptualisation of power, as productive, as creative, rather than restrictive and limiting, Mitchell Dean has synthesised some of the abovementioned writers' work to describe the practice of government as

> any more or less calculated and rational activity, undertaken by a multiplicity of authorities and agencies, employing a variety of techniques and forms of knowledge, that seeks to shape conduct by working through our desires aspirations, interests and beliefs, for definite but shifting ends and with a diverse set of relatively unpredictable consequences, effects and outcomes. (1999: 11)

Government is therefore not purely an array of technologies deployed by the state. Any practices that are concerned with directing the behaviour of individuals are understood as techniques of government. Therefore, we govern ourselves, others, institutions, discursive formations, non-discursive formations—the list is endless (Miller and Rose, 1990: 8). We can be articulated by others into the government of ourselves. Power is not understood as emanating purely from the state; it is conceived as passing through multiple sites, diffusing and transforming matter as it goes (Deleuze and Guattari, 1988: 224). States have simply become experts in exercising power, but they do not have ownership of it, as power is articulated rather then possessed (Deleuze, 1992: 60). Seeking to analyse the operation of power in this way emphasises how various technologies are operationalised to articulate a variety of strategies of government as the operation of 'intricate inter-dependencies between political rationalities and governmental technologies' (Rose and Miller, 1992: 176). Moreover, 'we can begin to understand the multiple and delicate networks that connect the lives of individuals, groups and organizations to the aspirations of authorities in the advanced liberal democracies of the present' (Rose and Miller, 1992: 176). Analysing the inter-dependencies between various technologies of government in making a particular programme realisable decentres the analysis of political power from its traditional object of the state (Deleuze, 1992: 22). Technologies can perform the tiniest of operations, but in assemblage they make realisable the most complex of political programmes.

While government is defined as the practice that describes the conducting of conduct, the term governmentality shall be used to describe something else:

> The term *governmentality* seeks to distinguish the particular mentalities, arts and regimes of government and administration that have emerged since 'early modern' Europe, while the term *government* is used as a more general term for any calculated direction of human conduct. (Dean, 1999: 2)

Governmentality is used to refer to particular rationalities of government concerned with organising or administrating particular populations. To study governmentality is to study the mentalities, or rationalities, of government, such as liberalism, social hygienism or conservatism. The study of governmentality attempts to describe the logic, ethics and opinions that make particular practices of government appear rational. To study governmentalities is to assert that the rationales that direct the 'conduct of conduct', through operationalising seemingly neutral technologies of power, need to be contextualised (Dean, 1999: 16). It is within this operationalising of mechanisms that otherwise appear to be neutral that allows for particular programmes of government to be so successful in acting upon two bodies: the population and the individual. A governmentality is not only a way of governing individuals, groups or spaces, it is always also a way of understanding them. It is a logic for how government should oper- ate, what sites it is justifiable for it to intervene upon and what the end goals of a group of activities are. Particular strategies of govern- ment use precise technologies to reveal the population in a specific fashion. The numerical underpinnings of many nineteenth-century governmentalities were discussed in Chapter 2. Elements that can be plotted numerically have attained high degrees of verity; they came to be considered as objective and factual, and their historicity became obscured. Perhaps this is related to mathematics' position as the most formalised of sciences. The move towards technologies of government that were numerical in their character resulted in many aspects of the machinery of government appearing scientific when they were still performing functions that were imbued with particular political and moral values (Ewald, 1990; Hacking, 1982, 1990, 1991; Miller, 2001). An analysis of government does not just study how these strategies are exercised, but also how these strategies have been formulated. A governmentality is the logic that makes particular strategies of govern- ment appear legitimate.

What is proposed is to analyse strategies of government. As they are deployed by the state, by schools, by individuals, '[a]n analytics of government attempts to show that our taken-for-granted ways of doing things and how we think about and question them are not entirely self-evident or necessary' (Dean, 1999: 21). Practices that are often left unquestioned are therefore problematised, as the particu- lar regimes for understanding and governing populations are inves- tigated. The interrelations between various branches of knowledge, dubious debates and political programmes are studied in an attempt to ask *how* we are governed. How we have become what we are. Dean (1999) summarises how such an analysis of government may depart with four 'how' questions:

1. characteristic forms of visibility, ways of seeing and perceiving
2. distinctive ways of thinking and questioning, relying on defi- nite vocabularies and procedures for the production of truth (e.g. those derived from the social, human and behavioural sciences)

3. specific ways of acting, intervening and directing, made up of particular types of practical rationality ('expertise' and 'know-how'), and relying upon definite mechanisms, techniques and technologies

4. characteristic ways of forming subjects, selves, persons, actors or agents (1999: 23)

Such '[a]n analytics of government examines the conditions under which regimes of practices come into being, are maintained and are transformed' (Dean, 1999: 21). The precise technological developments and changes described in Chapter 2 reorganised how the activity of government could take place. Strategies for governing particular aspects of the economy or activities conducted by certain groups were thus able to respond to the new technologies of power that had been developed. This created a feedback loop where technologies of power were being constructed to realise particular strategies of government. The existence of these new technologies of power generated new strategies of government in response to the new technological conditions.

An analytics of governmentality, as proposed by the theorists I have been discussing, rescinds from phrases such as 'the power of the state'. It is instead concerned with how and to what extent the state is articulated into the activity of government (Rose and Miller, 1992: 177). This process of articulating the machinery of the state into the activity of government is concerned with establishing what relations 'between political and other authorities; what funds, forces, persons, knowledge or legitimacy are utilised; and by means of what devices and techniques are these different tactics made operable' (Rose and Miller, 1992: 177). It is through this type of analysis that the diffusion of the political programmes of the state throughout society can be explained, but also the diffusion of political programmes that do not emanate from the state can be understood (Deleuze and Guattari, 1988: 214, 224).

An analysis of governmentality allows us to understand how the diffuse programmes, plans and political rationalities that have been articulated into the functioning of technologies of power became silently imbued with discreet political and moral values (Rose and Miller, 1992: 175). The functions of these technologies of power may be small, discreet and precise, but, acting in assemblage, these micro-operations significantly reformulate the population (Deleuze and Guattari, 1988: 398–9).

Government is a problematizing activity: it poses the obligations of rulers in terms of the problems they seek to address. The ideals of government are intrinsically linked to the problems around which it circulates, the failings it seeks to rectify, the ills it seeks to cure. Indeed the history of government might well be written as a history of problematizations, in which populations, intellectuals, philosophers, medics, military men, feminists and philanthropists have measured the real against the ideal and found it wanting. (Rose and Miller 1992: 181)

Government articulates relations of power to circulate around the body of the population. By problematising certain aspects of these bodies, some of these aspects may not even have been visible before power was articulated. Strategies of government concerned with proliferating certain attributes in bodies and managing the activities of groups, construct classifications to segment a population to further facilitate the precision of the activity of managing populations (Deleuze and Guattari, 1988: 211–13). As a problematising activity, government circulates onto the population, proliferating the problematics and ideas that justify its logic. It is through describing the way these strategies guide the articulation of power through particular technologies and onto distinct sites that the complex and diffuse way that power operates can be understood. It is in this way that the technical details of government can be described (Deleuze, 1992: 62; Foucault, 1979: 95–6). It is through the description of these technical details that strategies of government are analysed (Miller and Rose, 1990: 8).

In Chapter 2 I described the norm, statistics and intelligence tests as technologies of government or technologies of power. My definition of what these are derives from Rose and Miller:

Government is a domain of strategies, techniques and procedures through which different forces seek to render programmes operable, and by means of which a multitude of connections are established between the aspirations of authorities and the activities of individuals and groups. These heterogeneous mechanisms we term *technologies of government*. (1992: 183)

In a similar way to how Lazzarato (2002), and Rabinow and Rose (2006) have distinguished between bio-power and bio-politics (a distinction I have taken up in my research), it is necessary to establish what the conceptual differences are between a technology of power and a technology of government. A technology of power allows for power to flow in two directions. As power and resistance exist simultaneously, every technology has the potential to be used to facilitate flows of power or resistance. A technology of government will be used to refer to a technology of power that is being operationalised in the activity of government. A technology of power becomes a technology of government when it is utilised to achieve the goals of distinct rationalities or strategies. A number of technologies of power are typically operationalised by a strategy of government at the same time. Working in assemblage with one another they become a machinery of government concerned with purposefully achieving particular ends.

To engage in an analytics of government is to focus critical attention upon the manner in which the concerns and ambitions of those who sought to direct, manage and craft the lives of individuals have altered, depending upon what technologies they have at their disposal. It is technology that makes the activity of government possible (Dean, 1999: 31). Attention is focused upon analysing the invention and transformation of the apparatuses, mechanisms and devices whose purpose (or at least as a residual effect) shaped or directed the lives of individuals in some way. An analytics of government aims to unveil the connections between these procedures, practices and techniques, and wider political or moral programmes. These programmes represent strategies of government that, in turn, make up governmentalities (Dean, 1999: 16).

My analysis has thus far been concerned with describing how particular technological and economic developments altered how manageable the individual and the population were. The analysis of dyslexia I have undertaken largely takes place at the level of technologies of power, rather than strategies for governing populations.

I now want to describe how the invention of precise and multifaceted machineries of government affected particular strategies of government. The formation of these strategies of government occurred in a feedback loop, where these strategies were made possible by distinct technological developments generated by new technologies of government. This, in turn, made the goals of these emergent strategies of government increasingly realisable, allowing for complex strategies to be formulated. I will now turn my attention to proposing how strategies for governing reading began to respond to the increased reach of newly fashioned technologies of government.

The Mass Production of Texts

Texts, in principle, have always been reproducible. Since stone tablets were first engraved in ancient Mesopotamia it has been possible for a literate individual to copy and thus reproduce textual inscriptions. Before the invention of the printing press scribes were highly valued and would spend their lifetime copying books. For many years volumes upon volumes were copied by hand. It was, after all, the only way of reproducing a text. Clearly, the passages contained between the two covers had to be considered to be of great value if numerous individuals were to dedicate months, or even years, of their life to the reproduction of the same tome, as was the pursuit of monks copying works of religious scholarship. The value of the ability to read texts is implicit here. Reading gave an individual access to material of significant importance. Literate individuals were a crucial resource as they were able to reproduce the revered texts. The scarcity of these hand-copied texts made them coveted objects.

Gutenberg's invention of the printing press, sometime between 1450 and 1455, is often proclaimed to be the most important event in the history of reading (Childress, 2008). The ability to reproduce books cheaply and speedily, and distributing them among the population, altered our relationship with the written word forever. Books could now be produced mechanically. These were extremely different technical conditions to the reproduction of texts by hand. The invention of the printing press reduced the scarcity of books. In turn, this increase in the availability of texts changed the function that the book could perform. Over the centuries certain texts became more readily available, the Christian Bible being the most obvious example. The types of texts that inhabited the pages of books were transformed as the amount of time and effort required in its production diminished. The publication of texts that would previously have been seen as trivial could now be justified. As time progressed, books became less concerned with religious or other suitably lofty matters, with whole literary genres being invented that were inconceivable before this technological innovation. The popular publishing industry was born and an avalanche of reading matter began that has yet to suffer an abeyance.

Readers—individuals able to comprehend inscription—have long been reproducible. One literate subject is able to pass this skill on to another. While this process is as old as the first alphabet, the intent to inscribe this skill onto not just individual bodies but the body of the population is a relatively recent occurrence. It is with the introduction of mass education that technologies of government began to articulate bio-power and thus actively produce a literate population (Hunter, 1988). As it became necessary to produce a population with a certain degree of literacy, schools and a variety of other programmes concerned with spreading literacy were thus articulated into the activity of government (Procacci, 1978: 55).

With these changes in both the production and government of texts and readers, concurrent changes occurred in how texts and readers were conceived of. The activity of reading was transformed at a technological level. Texts have been diffused throughout society, becoming a part of how we make money, enjoy ourselves; how we learn to do both mundane tasks and develop complex ideas. Reading has not just proliferated throughout the population, its place in our day-to-day life has ameliorated. In response to this transformation of reading, the type of texts being produced has multiplied, expanded and become refashioned as the potential for texts to become conduits through which information is received, or containers providing instructions for performing a particular task, was realised. I will now describe how this way of conceiving of the activity of reading and viewing a text is a departure from how they were considered prior to their mass production. I shall undertake this through a discussion of various histories of reading, literature and schooling the shifting styles of governing reading.

Governing the Danger of Literacy Through Limitation

At our current juncture, where the production of texts has become digital and literacy is common place, it is easy to forget the place that the written word, and the activity of reading, holds in the three great Abrahamic religions. With both the ability to read and physical texts being scarce during the formation of these religions, the social position of reading would, of course, have been quite different to how it is now. This veneration of the book and reading is repeated across the writings of scientists, authors and statesmen, deriving, perhaps, from the place they hold in these religions (Derrida, 1997: 16). I shall attempt to review a variety of literature that can inform this argument. A particular emphasis shall be placed upon metaphors connected to the activity of reading. Below I attempt to describe, through a review of histories of reading and literature, where this historical metaphor is discussed.

Alberto Manguel's *History of Reading* has been particularly important in reviewing the way that the activity of reading has altered. I will begin by quoting Manguel's description of how the activity of reading and the text were extolled in the Jewish and Christian traditions:

The universe in, Judaeo-Christian tradition, is conceived of as a written Book made from numbers and letters; the key to understanding the universe lies in our ability to read these properly and master their combination, and thereby learn to give life in some part of the colossal text, in imitation of our Maker. (According to a fourth-century legend, the Talmudic scholars Hanani and Hshaiah would once a week study the *Sefer Yezirah* and, by the right combination of letters, create a three-year-old calf which they would have for dinner) (1997: 8).

In Islam, this notion is extended. Not only is the Koran one of God's many creations, it is also one of his attributes. In Jewish and Christian antiquity reading was thus considered to be a powerful process. Reading the word of God allowed one to come unspeakably close to God and His infinite truth. Through reading religious texts one was considered to be capable of understanding the truth about the world. The story of Hannai and Hshaiah above suggests that there was understood to be a correspondence between the scriptures and the world. The secrets of God's earthly creation are to be found through the devoted, precise and persistent study of scripture. In the Abrahamic tradition reading becomes an activity imbued with religious significance. Careful, meticulous, scholarly study of religious text was thus revered as one of the most holy practices in these faiths. The world is a book written by God, the meaning of which man was tasked with unravelling.

The art of interpretation—hermeneutics—was born out of biblical scholarship. Precise reverential understanding of the text was needed. The word of God needed to be understood to the best of our ability. Reading was an art. An art mastered by the holy. To understand the world was to read it. As Mieke Bal (2005) recounts, the art of interpretation was not restricted to texts in the strictest sense: stained glass windows were also interpreted by priests *as* texts. A congregation that could not collectively read the Bible was thus able to read stained glass windows together, as guided by the sermons of priests. Here '[t]he image does not replace the text; it *is* one' (Bal, 2005: 35). The activity of reading with its relation to the Abrahamic heritage of discovering truths of the world through careful scholarship made relating to any object, textual or not, an act of reading. Scientific researchers have often seen their research as an attempt to read the great book of nature, re-animating this metaphor (Derrida, 1997: 16). Here, the scholar is using a different set of tools to facilitate his/her reading, and the object being read is understood as being ultimately textual—once the complex language of nature has been mastered it is possible to read the world. This metaphor's centrality to our ideas of scholarship has no doubt directed the character and direction of scientific research, practices of government and the arts.

A discussion of this metaphor has an important place in one of Jacques Derrida's first projects, *Of Gramatology*, which begins with a consideration of the importance of the foundation of this metaphor for western metaphysics.[2] He begins by stating:

> There remains to be written a history of this metaphor, a metaphor that systematically contrasts a divine or natural writing and human and laborious finite and artificial inscription. It remains to articulate rigorously the stages of that history as marked by the quotations below, and to follow the theme of God's book (nature or law, indeed natural law) through all its modifications. (1997: 15)

For Derrida this metaphor is absolutely foundational for Western theology, philosophy and science. It is through recourse to the book of nature that it has been possible for these endeavours, as we know them, to develop. While Derrida is not trying to devalue the achievements of these disciplines, or their ability to operate—it is clear after all that scientific research is often able to describe complex phenomena with high degrees of exactitude–he is simply alerting his readers to the presence of this metaphor at the core, and its unquestioned status. His deconstruction here is not seeking to destroy. He suggests that the metaphor privileges originary or divine writing, and consequently devalues the writing of men as inferior or corrupted. An array of quotations is then presented by scholars of all kinds to reinforce the importance of this metaphor. I have reproduced them here as they direct our attention to the privileged and poetic way that reading was conceived in the strategy of limitation, with the majority of the quotations originating before literacy became commonplace:

> Rabbi Eliezer said 'If all the seas were of ink, and all ponds planted with reeds, if the sky and the earth were parchments and if all human beings practised the art of writing—they would not exhaust the Torah I have learned just as the Torah itself would not be diminished any more than is the sea by the water removed by a pain brush dipped in it'.

Galileo: 'It [the book of Nature] is written in a mathematical language'.

Descartes: '... To read in the great book of Nature...'.

Dema, in the name of natural religion, in the *Dialogues*...of Hume: 'And this volume of nature contains a great an inexplicable riddle, more than any intelligible discourse or reasoning'.

Bonnet: 'It would seem more philosophical to me to presume that our earth is a book that God has given to intelligences far superior to ours to read, and where they study in depth the infinitely multiple and varied characters of His adorable wisdom'.

G.H. von Schubert: 'This language made of images and hieroglyphs, which supreme Wisdom uses in all its revelations to humanity— which is found in the inferior [*nieder*] language of poetry—and which, in the most inferior and imperfect way [*auf der allerniedrigsten und unvollkommensten*], is more like the metaphorical expression of the dream than the prose of wakefulness...we may wonder if this language is not the true and wakeful language of the superior regions. If, when we consider ourselves, awakened we are not plunged in a millennial slumber, or at least in the echo of its dreams, where we only perceive a few isolated and obscure words of God's language, as a sleeper perspectives the conversation of the people around him'.

Jaspers: 'This word is the manuscript of an other, inaccessible to a universal reading which only existence deciphers'. (1997: 16)

Derrida discusses how the same metaphor is at work in the above texts, arguing that an originary writing is being posited. This writing is truthful because it is original, it proceeds man and is divine. Human writing is secondary and inferior to this writing of a divine origin. For Derrida this is symptomatic of the rationalism of Western metaphysics. The rationality of Western theology, science and philosophy depends on this metaphor, from which they derive perspectives on truth. The truth made by men is only an attempt to understand the originary truth of God. Derrida then develops this into an argument where speech is the originary writing given by God to man, and inscription is inferior—man made. Writing in the form of inscriptions upon tablets, parchments or paper is therefore too secondary and inferior. His argument then builds upon this by describing how this exclusion is necessary for the development of Jean-Jacques Rousseau's thought and subsequently the anthropology of Claude Lévi-Strauss.

Derrida's reading of the quotations, despite its skill, erudition and inventiveness, takes place at the expense of an alternate, or perhaps a concurrent, reading where the place of *reading* in these quotes is not diminished or excluded (reading is considered only three times in *Of Grammatology*). Reading is venerated in the above quotations as the process by which the historical truth of God or nature is accessed. Reading is, of course, the process by which this divine writing is accessed. Reading is, however, almost absent in Derrida's analysis. So, while an originary text is being presupposed, Derrida does not consider the distinct ability of some individuals to access this text through study. These fragments seem to be as much about the importance of being able to read this divine originary text as the presupposed existence of this divine text. Reading is conceived here as a way of accessing immortal timeless truths, gaining access to God, or the secret of his creation. The act of reading is being positioned as the most potent activity an individual can engage in.

Historically, many groups have been, and indeed still are, restricted in their access to books or the ability to learn to read (this will be discussed in some depth later in the chapter). While in some sites this strategy of limitation remained (and it is unlikely that it will ever completely disappear), as strategies of government became more concerned with fostering the populations' abilities, and as the population became increasingly capitalised, the needs that the economy required of the individual body changed concurrently, and a new strategy of governing reading formed and became prevalent (for a discussion of the relationship between the capitalisation of the population and the economy see Foucault (1979, 2007, 2010) and Chapter 2). This strategy was concerned with developing subjects who were literate enough to engage in the more complex tasks that their employment required of them (Jones and Williamson, 1979). Many jobs that, on first glance, may not appear to require literacy are, in fact, reliant upon skills that would have been developed through reading or the good habits that many of schoolmasters believed would be imbued into bodies by teaching them how to read. This strategy involved the proliferation of a particular attribute—a strategy that would seem to be complimentary to the move from sovereign power to bio-power (Foucault, 1979: 135–43).

It would be wrong, however, to consider reading as referring to the same activity in both strategies. The strategy of proliferation is concerned with assembling the body so that it is hospitable to the transmission of necessary knowledge. Reading becomes one of the ways of producing conduits through which power can flow and a more useful body can be sculpted, managed and shaped. The potential of reading to imbue a morality in the population was also realised in this strategy (Hunter, 1988; Jones and Williamson, 1979; Viswanathan, 1989: 20). Reading, in the strategy of limitation, is limited because of the potential power that readers can articulate. Although their potential access to eternal truth is no doubt essential to the arts of governing, science and art itself, these subjects also pose a danger to the states they inhabit. Here, the increased economic potential of a literate population does not offset the increased dangers that a literate population poses. As the precision of technologies of government increased it became apparent that these same powers could be articulated to proliferate moral attributes throughout a particular population, and through this some of the dangers of literate population could be managed (Hunter, 1988; Jones and Williamson, 1979; Viswanathan, 1989).

The Proliferation of Texts and the Proliferation of Readers

Today we read texts with less reverence. Texts now often function as a container of information. If the invention of the printing press generated an avalanche of texts, then the twentieth century, with the advent of digital texts, has been a literary tsunami that only appears to be intensifying. We are in contact with texts constantly: receipts; notice boards; instruction booklets; newspapers; novels; emails; signposts; blogs; graffiti. The online interactive encyclopaedia *Wikipedia* now has more than four million articles. We read this mammoth array of texts constantly, rarely reflecting upon the activity that we are engaged in. The activity of reading rarely holds the spiritual connotation it did in the Abrahamic religions for Descartes or Gallieo (Derrida, 1997: 16; Manguel, 1997: 8). Reading today is rarely an act where some sort of divine truth is accessed; it is today a means of receiving information. Benedictine monks were instructed to hold, 'if possible', the books they read 'in their left hands, wrapped in the sleeve of their tunics and resting on their knees; their right hands shall be uncovered with which to grip and turn the pages' (Manguel, 1997: 15). Books are no longer treated with this degree of care; they are no longer surrounded by such carefully constructed rituals, unless, of course, their age and scarcity has imbued them with high monetary value. In its every day instantiation reading has lost its ritualism, its prestige; it is less of an art and more of a technique (Manguel, 1997: 281). Reading is perceived as a means to an end, rather than a poetic activity.

While the invention of the printing press changed how the written word was thought of forever, there is an event that must be considered to be of equal or greater importance in the history of reading. That event is, of course, the billions of readers that have been produced since the introduction of mass education. Reading and the book have undergone dramatic changes in how they are perceived; the object once venerated is now commonplace and often a stale container of information. Reading, a skill once only possessed by the few, is now possessed by the many. Reading is no longer the art it once was to Talmudic scholars, Benedictine monks or even nineteenth-century British gentlemen—it is now reduced to a banal attribute that we are all expected to acquire in our youth. If this technological conception of reading has become dominant at the expense of an artistic conception, the importance of the activity of reading has not diminished. In fact, its importance to strategies of government has augmented. The increased regularity with which we engage with texts has increased the importance of reading not just for government, but also for the governed. The ability to read texts is now expected of the majority of the population—those who have difficulty reading are therefore problematised. I will now describe initial British debates on the topic of mass education. My intent is to show how a shift from a strategy of limiting literacy to one of proliferating literate bodies was achieved.

In 1807 a series of parliamentary debates on education began. The series started with a bill proposed by Samuel Whitbread, dealing with the poor law (Hansard, 24 April, 1807, pp. 538–50). The bill suggested that the parish should be responsible for the education of its children, and that a child should have two years of compulsory education that would be administrated between the ages of seven and fourteen years. It was hoped that education would reduce crime and reduce pauperism (Hansard, 24 April, 1807, pp. 538–50). Compulsory education was therefore being suggested, not out of a moral need, but to facilitate the production of a more desirable population. Its rationale was bio-political, disciplinary in its character. For many ministers there was no need for the poor to be educated; it could, in fact, be dangerous. Mr Rose stated he had 'no doubt, that the poor ought to be taught to read', but regarding 'writing, he had some doubt, because those who had learnt to write well were not willing to abide at the plough, but looked to a situation in some counting house' (Hansard, 24 April, 1807, pp. 538–50). Rose feared that mass education would produce individuals that wished to aspire beyond their place in society, finding their work unfulfilling.

Even advocates of the bill, such as Sharpe, expressed support by describing the positive affects it would have on the bodies of individuals:

> ...though they should forget all their learning, would have collected many beneficial habits of indelible nature; habits of submission and respect for their superiors; habits of cleanliness and exertion and the fear of punishment. (Hansard, 24 April, 1807, pp. 538–50)

Sharpe supported mass education so that 'unruly masses' would be reshaped from a dangerous disrespecting rabble, to an obedient population (Hansard, 24 April, 1807, pp. 538–50). The possible economic benefits of refiguring the population through the deployment of an educational machinery calibrated to articulate disciplinary power seems to be the primary axis of the debate.

In 1807 the Lord of the Manor of Barton founded a school for forty poor children; the intent was considered to be charitable. Instruction given by Lord Barton elucidates his worries of the danger education could bring: 'All children are to be taught to read but none are to be taught the dangerous arts of writing or arithmetic except such as the Lord of the manor shall think fit' (Barton quoted in Rich, 1970: 16). Lord Barton was concerned with providing the moral instruction that would make 'good Christians' and workers out of the children, but he was also distressed about working class children gaining middle class skills and attributes. Texts were to be deployed as moralising technologies, but it was feared that a literate population could be an unruly population. Reading and writing were considered to be dangerous as they encouraged critical thinking. The essence of reading, after all, is reflection. As Franz Kafka remarked to a friend, 'One reads in order to ask questions' (Kafka quoted in Glatzer, 1974: 53). Reading engenders questioning and, of course, when someone becomes a questioner, they realise that no voice is infallible. Those individuals who were granted the right to a literate education had to be limited. Those who governed populations assessed the implications of proliferating literacy amongst the bodies they governed. British slave owners were one such group that was concerned that if literacy spread amongst the enslaved population they

> might find dangerous revolutionary ideas in books. They did not believe those who argued that a literacy restricted to the Bible would strengthen the bonds of society; they realized that if slaves could read the Bible, they could also read abolitionist tracts, and that even

in the Scriptures the slaves might find inflammatory notions of revolt and freedom. (Manguel, 1997: 279–80).

While the potential benefits of a moralising a population of enslaved people were recognised, the dangers presented too great a risk to the plantation owners. The danger of fostering the skill of reading in a population, without proper religious instruction, was also identified in a report by the Select Committee of 1816 Education of the Lower Orders in the Metropolis:

> Q. Do you think any danger is to be apprehended by giving children knowledge, without communicating religious ideas?
>
> A. Certainly there is danger: because you give them information and a greater power, without at the same time a principle to direct that power. (1816: 495)

If a population is equipped with the ability to read then it is understood to have the potential to direct relations of power that they would previously not have been able to articulate. A literate individual has access to a greater number of capillaries of power than a non-literate individual (Manguel, 1997: 281). The concern here is that without religious instruction to provide moral guidance these relations of power would be articulated in a way that did not fit with the interest of the most dominant governmentality. Jones and Williamson (1979) allude to some of the relations of power that can be accessed by literate individuals: 'A class was defined in part... [by] the type of literature they read and peculiarities of their language' (Jones and Williamson, 1979: 81). Access to particular vocabularies, knowledge and culture allowed access to particular spaces, institutions and, ultimately, technologies of power.

The dangers of educating a population were being articulated as if the population was capital. Interests and pursuits that the labourers would not find already present in their manual work must not be fostered. Lord John Russell, aware of the economic need to educate the population, alerted the house to his fears:

> ...so far from being afraid of instruction, the only question in men's minds was, whether the National Schools were not too highly instructing the people—whether, in regard to the portion of the people who were engaged in outdoor manual occupations, they were not educating them to the prejudice of their physical capacity. (Hansard, 22 May, 1851, p. 1279)

Minsters were incredibly concerned about the ability of working class children to be economically useful after they had undertaken a certain degree of a specific type of education.

The Elementary Education Act of 1870 did not introduce free or compulsory education. However, it did establish many of the conditions for its implementation. The level of state involvement with education increased dramatically. The state was still concerned with the production of bodies, but the type of body that the government wished to craft had changed. Industry increasingly required an educated populace and we have seen, thus far, reading had been deployed as the main strategy both for educating children and introducing them to moral and ethical ideas hospitable to the needs of industry.

Technologies of Proliferation 1: The School

The object of every system of education for the working classes especially, ought to be *the infusion of Christian principles, and at the same time the cultivation of Christian habits.* Now the question is, have schools actually the machinery or platform for accomplishing both? Have our schools the covered and uncovered rooms? Have they the convenient school-room and convenient enclosed play-ground, and is the maser a superintendent in both? Do our schools instil good principles, and if they do so, do they also cultivate good habits? We answer that the improved intellectual system embraces the former, but makes no provision for the latter; indeed we are shut up to the conclusion that we have no schools but those for infant training, and those formed after the same system, which cultivate *the child*, or train him when not under the eyes of his parents 'in the way he should go.' Infant training is unquestionably the primary and most powerful moral lever of society, because it commences before bad habits can have been formed, *'beginning at the beginning'* (Stow, 1836: 18, original emphasis)

Karen Jones and Kevin Williamson's *The Birth of the Schoolroom* (1979) is one of the first attempts to operationalise the Foucauldian approach to historical questions onto a new surface, and is still one of the most successful attempts at doing so. They describe a shift in nineteenth-century British educational manuals from the intent to teach useful habits, such as cleanliness, good time-keeping and the production of a more literate population, to a strategy of pedagogic production where the moralisation of bodies is the paramount concern. While I broadly agree with Jones and Williamson, I would contend that it bears the mark of being an early Foucauldian study, as economic issues are somewhat sidelined.[3] The non-discursive formation of the economy's influence in establishing bodies with a certain kind of literacy goes un-witnessed by Jones and Williamson.

The move Jones and Williamson (1979) describe, from the production of docile bodies to moralised bodies, is, to me, not an epistemological break[4] in a strategy of government, but the strategy's intensification as the potency of the technologies of power that had been assembled to educate the populations becomes evident. The technologies of power assembled as the school, as the entire educational system, can, if calibrated correctly, reach far deeper into the body of the population than was first imagined. This forms part of a process by which relations of power became increasingly microscopic in their focus. Technologies of power were now able to reach sites hitherto considered ungovernable and, in some cases, previously invisible. This process characterises the development of bio-politics throughout the nineteenth and twentieth centuries.

Jones and Williamson describe how, in addition to imbuing bodies with particular skills and attributes, the school also performed a taxonomic function. It became a crucial site in the arrangement, organisation and classification of bodies:

> The guiding principles of this 'intellectual organ' were the division of labour, mutual instruction, classification, minute discipline, constant surveillance and ceaseless activity. The school existed as a finely calibrated disciplinary machine for the arrangement and classification of bodies, and the promotion and regulation of preferred activities. (1979: 73)

As the school became increasingly geared to classifying bodies, a feedback loop was established between the non-discursive formation of the school and the medical sciences; the school offered a site where the taxonomists of medicine could experiment (Rose, 1985). The existence of this space of taxonomic experimentation allowed for the imagination of medical classification to augment. As has been discussed in the last chapter, the development of the school took place concurrently with the reorganisation of life around the poles of normal and abnormal, and the measuring of a populations' attributes by statistics (Ewald, 1990, 1991; Hacking, 1982, 1990). The population of a school could be studied and segmented into smaller populations, and could be acted upon with a previously unavailable precision. The school provided one of the key sites during the nineteenth century where relations of bio-power were to be articulated through a carefully assembled and pre-cisely calibrated machinery of government (Procacci, 1978: 55). These developments, and the creation of precise technologies of measurement such as intelligence tests, all played a significant part in establishing the population of a school as a body with divergent attributes that needed to be carefully managed to meet its full potential. Rose (1985) describes how the psychology of the individual utilised the school as the main site to establish its disciplinary machinery, how the school and indi-vidual psychology were necessary for each others' development.

Jones and Williamson describe how Bell's Madras (Bell, 1813) system allowed for the activity of classification and teaching to be calibrated so that they complimented one another. This is a key example of how an array of technologies of power were finely tuned and carefully organised to make realisable the goals of a particular rationality of government:

> The classification of the pupils and the matter to be learned made possible by the calibration of the two, and the emergence of practices accountability—the charting of the daily, weekly and yearly pro-gress. Under the Madras system, the pupil 'every day puts down in his books the day of the month, at the termination of his day's task. And, on a page at the end of his book, he daily registers the number of lessons said, pages written, sums thought, etc.'. (Bell, 1813: 16 in Jones and Williamson, 1979: 74)

These systems had a dual function; not only did they allow for con-trol and surveillance, but they also allowed for the collection of know-ledge about the young (Jones and Williamson 1979: 74). Jones and Williamson quote Bell, describing how the systems operated: 'In the hands of the master the registers are instruments of discipline, and pro-duce great precision and exactitude, enabling him readily to inspect, direct, conduct and controul [sic] the respective classes' (Bell, 1813: 18). The ultimate aims of elementary education, as a variety of technologies of power articulated into the activity of government, are presented by Jones and Williamson through a quotation from Bell:

> …good subjects, good men, good Christians, for which the machin-ery of the school constituted the appropriate means. To attain these ends…the grand desideratum is to fix attention, to call forth exer-tion, to prevent the waste of time in school. This, in the madras

school, is achieved, not by vulgar and coarse instruments which reach no further than the body, and produce only a degrading and momentary effect, but by the strong and permanent hold which its machinery takes of the mind, and the deep impression, which it makes on the heart. (1813: preface)

The bio-political character of this particular machinery of government is further illustrated in a quotation from the educational campaigner Bernard: 'it provides for their education and prepares them for their course through life by early habits of ORDER, CLEANILNESS AND APPLICATION' (Bernard, 1809: 203–4, original emphasis). Initially, technologies of government that articulated bio-power directed power in a disciplinary character. However, they became fully bio-political when they ceased to predominately limit behaviours and took on the additional operation of proliferating desirable behaviours throughout the population, producing a certain kind of literate body, spreading good habits, like good time-keeping and cleanliness. The school operated as a panoptic machine. The main character of power relations that were articulated through this carefully calibrated machine was, at this point, disciplinary. As the '[s]tatements on the need for popular education at the beginning of the nineteenth century were made in relation to the problem of reducing the expense of poor relief, while at the same time maintaining the welfare of the labouring power' (Jones and Williamson, 1979: 63). Techniques such as '[s]elf-instruction under surveillance was both a model of discipline and order, and an engine of self-improvement and beneficial activity' (Jones and Williamson, 1979: 73). The shift that Jones and Williamson describe (from disciplining bodies to make sure they had good time-keeping and cleanliness to moralising populations) illustrates how strategies of government became more ambitious in their goals. Attributes, expertise and a variety of human characteristics could now be fostered that would previously been seen to be beyond the technical abilities that were at the disposal of schools. As the machinery of the school developed, it could be fine-tuned to perform a more complex function: the proliferation of moral values throughout the student body.

Jones and Williamson (1979) describe how the interior of the school was designed to facilitate these new, increasingly complex functions that the school had acquired, governing attributes previously considered ungovernable:

The new objective for popular education, which was definitive of its necessity in this period, gave rise to a new set of problems concerning the interior space of the school. The school was now defined as a machinery of moral training, rather than as an engine of instruction. There was a change in the rules governing the design of the machinery of the school, which corresponded to this change in function, involving a redefinition of the role of the teacher within this machinery, and changes in the definition of the aims and character of pedagogic practice. (1979: 87)

The recognition that teachers were equipped with necessary expertise and specialised attributes to be a part of this more complex assemblage of government illustrates that technologies of power were invented to respond to the population, as re-modelled by a previous array of technologies of power (Jones and Williamson, 1979: 87). The machinery of the school was initially constructed to facilitate the operation of disciplinary power. As the bio-political functions of this machinery were realised, the operation of schools in this assemblage was recalibrated in relation to this reoriented strategy of government. Jones and Williamson describe the recalibration of the machinery of schooling towards the goal of proliferating moral values throughout a population:

Whereas the main objective of the monitorial system was to teach children reading, writing and the elements of religion and thereby form principles of conduct and useful habits, by contrast the training systems advocated by Stow, Kay-Shuttleworth, Symons and Carpenter, had as their main aims the formation or reformation of a set of dispositions within children, and a development of their moral intellectual and practical understanding, useful dispositions being, for example, a love of one's brother man, a love of knowledge, a love of cleanliness, a love of labour, and a love of order. And it was precisely through the relationship to the teacher that these aims were to be achieved. (1979: 88)

Instilling in the population the ability to read imbued them with the ability to become more moral, but risked giving them access to a new variety of capillaries of resistance. The ambitions of strategies of governing populations of school children had augmented owing to technical advancement.

Technologies of Proliferation 2: English Literature

Gauri Viswanathan's *Masks of Conquest* shows that the invention of the discipline of English literature in India cannot be separated from the colonial machinery of government and the specific goals of educating and civilising colonial subjects. She argues that boundaries of the subject itself were formed to further the administrative and political objectives of British colonial rule in India, and posits that English literature was invented as a scholarly concern in the colonies before its study began upon British soil. Viswanathan's description of how the discipline of English literature operated in India, explains why it was invented in India before its study began in Great Britain. Humanistic functions were associated with the study of literature: 'for example, the shaping of character or development of the aesthetic sense or the disciplines of ethical thinking—were considered essential to the processes of socio-political control by the guardians of the same tradition' (Viswanathan, 1989: 3). Viswanathan's description of how the study of English literature was utilised to proliferate a set of moral values throughout the Indian population illustrates how the government of reading has been articulated into the government of the population in a variety of different ways. For Viswanathan the introduction of English literatures marks

> the effacement of sordid history of colonialist expropriation, material exploitation, and class and race oppression behind European dominance. The English literary text, functioning as a surrogate Englishman in his highest and most perfect state, becomes a mask for economic exploitation, so successfully camouflaging the material activities of the colonizer that one unusually self-conscious British Colonial official, Charles Trevelyan, was prompted to remark '[The Indians] daily converse with the best and wisest Englishmen through the medium of their works, and from perhaps higher idea of our nation than if the intercourse with it were of a more personal kind'. (1989: 20)

The invention of English literature as an academic discipline shows that there was immense confidence in the ability of technologies of power to be articulated in the activity of government. The articulation of the literary text in the activity of government in colonial India is a similar operation to that which mass schooling took on in the UK, where it became concerned with proliferating a set of moral values into the body of the population (Hunter, 1998; Jones and Williamson, 1979). With the English literary text propounding a set of aesthetic and moral values, it came to act as a surrogate Englishman. Deploying literary texts in the activity of government articulated government in a less visible way. A canon of texts looks less like the machinery of government than armed men, ambassadors and policy decrees. An assemblage of government was formed concerned with proliferating values that were amenable to a particular governmentality. This assemblage was able to act in a way that appeared not to be dominating. The reasoning proclaimed for the teaching of English and the function it eventually performed were quite different:

> A discipline that was originally introduced in India primarily to con-vey the mechanics of language was thus transformed into an instru-ment for ensuring industriousness, efficiency, trustworthiness, and compliance in native subjects. (Viswanathan, 1989: 93)

The reading of texts from foreign canons provoked grave concern from the colonial rulers. The British administration was more concerned about the reading of Goethe than the reading of political liberals such as Locke or Hume. The German romantic tradition was feared as poten-tially forming a unified national sentiment through the transmission of 'dangerous values' to the educated Indian populace. Nationalist writers such as Bengali novelist Rankin Chandra Chatterjee attempted to revive the myths of their people in order to proliferate a differ-ent set of values amongst the population (Viswanathan, 1989: 157). Establishing a literate population and drawing attention to literature's moralising potentials became an extremely dangerous proposition for those engaged in the activity of government. There was concern that the literate education of the Indians would affect their economic productivity:

> ...writers like the Bengali novelist Rankin Chandra Chatterjee, who were schooled in the best Western literary establishments in Bengal, turned their attention to reviving myths and tales of the past to stir up longing in the people for a return of a golden age. Maine's allusion to the spirit of reconstruction of a Roman literary model of German Romanticism. The fact that the educated Indians were reading Goethe in translation caused infinitely greater con-cern in British administrative circles than their reading the works of political liberals Locke or Hume, whose appeal to reason and

constitutionalism rather than the imagination presumably posed fewer dangers of shaping a unified nationalist sentiment. (Viswanathan, 1989: 157)

While the ability to read approved British writers who would have been seen to instil values that were in the interests of the activity of government was considered to be of utility, there was another consequence. A literate Indian population could now also access a canon which contained values antithetical to the goals of government. Making visible the moral values that many literary texts contained allowed for capillaries of resistance to be deployed in opposition to the activity of government. The articulation of the study of literature into the activity of government diffused colonial rule therefore changing the style of government in India. However, it also bought with it a new set of risks.

One of these risks was the tension created between:

> ...the upward mobility by modern studies and the limited opportunities open to the colonized for advancement exposed the fundamental paradox of British imperialism: economic exploitation required the sanction of higher motives, but once colonial intervention took on a moral justification—that is, the improvement of a benighted people—the pressure to sustain the expectations of the people by an equalization of educational opportunities created new internal stresses. Nothing less than the most extraordinary political agility was called for in reconciling capitalist system of production to flourish. The price of failure of course was the exposure of the moral pretensions of British colonialism. At one level, education as part of the state is complicit with the reproduction of an economic and cultural order. But because education is also expected to provide opportunities for advancement, it becomes an arena of social conflict, and the tension ultimately reduced the British administration to a position of acute vulnerability and paralysis. (Viswanathan 1989: 164)

The introduction of literary studies in India helped to transform the body of the population; a strategy of proliferating literacy had inadvertently made some of the strategies it had been designed to facilitate harder to achieve. Educating the Indian middle classes in English literature paradoxically produced subjects both technically and morally amenable to the goals of the British rulers, but also imbued the subjects with a variety of moral values that furthered the possible base for insurrection, as the opportunities promised in the values that had been instilled with were not always available. The concerns appear to be similar to those of the select committee of 1816. The study of English literature was a moralising activity; the same skills of reading could be operationalised to read literature that did not adhere to the colonists plans to develop reasons to resist. A literate population poses a different set of challenges to those who govern an illiterate one (Manguel, 1997: 281).

Ian Hunter's *Culture and Government* is a genealogy of literary education. It too is concerned, like Viswanathan, with the invention of English literature and its relationship to particular rationales of government. Hunter's genealogy is divided into two halves: a study of the emergence of mass schooling and the development of literary criticism. For Hunter the emergence of English literature takes place during a period when:

> ...an historically unprecedented machinery of social investigation and investigation and administration, which began to emerge in England during the late nineteenth century and which by the middle of the nineteenth had largely succeeded in constituting the life of the population as an object of government. (1988: ix)

Hunter's argument draws upon Foucault and situates these developments in a similar framework to the governmentality literature I have discussed above. Viswanathan's (1989) and Hunter 's (1988) research shows how the codification of culture articulated a vast array of cultural products into the activity of government.

Conclusion

This chapter has suggested that reading has always been intensively governed: who could read; what sort of texts they came into contact with; the level of the interpretative skills that were encouraged; whether they were taught the associated arts of writing and arithmetic; the aspirations they were taught to associate with their newly acquired skills; the level of association they were permitted to have with dangerous foreign canons. These, it was thought, could imbue a population with feared foreign values. Reading was intensively governed because it allowed for the articulation of productive relations of power. It has been argued that during a shift from a sovereign style of government to a liberal bio-politics, the manner by which reading was governed also altered. A strategy of limiting the amount of literate bodies was replaced by a strategy of proliferating literacy throughout the population. A variety of technologies were developed concerned with proliferating literacy, such as the school. This shift in the style of government not only changed the strategy of how reading should be governed, or the precise minutia of technologies that governed reading (which, of course, multiplied and dispersed); the rationality changed as it had now become politically useful to have numerous literate or semi-literate people in the population.

For the state, a problem was thus posed: a literate population was needed, owing to the complex nature of the economy, but the ability to read, as has been recounted above, had long been feared by those who were concerned with the conduct of conduct as a deeply dangerous attribute. I find resonance in Manguel's words once again: 'As centuries of dictators have known, an illiterate crowd is easiest to rule; since the craft of reading cannot be untaught once it has been acquired, the second-best recourse is to limit its scope' (Manguel, 1997: 281). States deploy educational institutions to equip the population with the craft of reading, not the dangerous art. Reading is proliferated as a technique for receiving information, rather than an art that allows for discovery. A technique stripped of all the potency associated with the activity in Islam, the Jewish Torah (Manguel, 1997: 8), or the great philosophers, theologians and scientists (Derrida, 1997: 16). A different kind of literacy was being proliferated throughout the population; it was less of an art and more of a technique. It was, however, still a precarious pursuit for governments to attempt to equip their population with the technique of reading. As is known from Heidegger, technology and art have the same origin; the technique of reading always has the potential to become the dangerous art (Heidegger, 1977: 34). Imbuing a population with literacy has long caused those concerned with governing to fret (Hunter, 1989; Manguel, 1989: 281; Viswasnathan, 1989).

The disparate technologies and distinct rationalities of government that intersected to produce dyslexia now need to be described. The emergence of a strategy of proliferating literacy should be understood as related to a shift from a governmentality that deployed sovereign power to those that predominately articulated relations of bio-power. Foucault (1979), Rose (1991, 1993, 1999), Dean (1999) and Hacking (1982) have described how politics had become a 'bio-politics', whereby both the body of the population and the body of the individual had become capitalised as they became resources to be cultivated through intervention. This capitalisation of the population facilitated a shift in how the population was to be considered and how it could be acted upon. Specific technologies of government were constructed that facilitated the development of a strategy of producing a literate population, such as compulsory schooling; the norm; psychological sciences; intelligence tests, both general and attribute-specific. A feedback loop exists here between rationalities of government and technologies of power. Shifts in governmentality affected the production of particular technologies of power. In turn, these technologies of power caused strategies of government to realign and reshape as their goals developed in response to new operations that were made possible by the recently constructed technologies of power. Dyslexia is being posited here as a specific technology of power that facilities the flowing of power onto and through specific bodies; a technology of power that is made possible after the refiguration of the body of the individual and the body of the population.

This book will now consider dyslexia as a technology of power, one that, in turn, facilitates a variety of strategies of governing reading. The invention, ossification and operation of dyslexia as a technology for facilitating power relations will now be described.

4
Reading Difficulties Become a Medical Concern

Having difficulty with reading, or being unable to read, has not always been a medical problem. In the late nineteenth century, physicians such as Broadbent (1872) and Hinshelwood (1895) became interested in identifying particular bodies with reading difficulties. These physicians were able to establish a particular population of persons understood as having reading difficulties. This chapter is focused around the question of 'how' reading difficulties were invented as a concern for medical researchers. I describe how this interest began to solidify into a diagnostic category, leading them to write reports in some of the most well-known and respected medical journals in Britain (Hinshelwood, 1895; Kussmaul, 1877). In response to this problem I will consider how the diagnosis of acquired word-blindness, a technology of power, was crafted, paying particular attention to why a difficulty with reading, in its acquired form, became a medical concern during the late nineteenth century. It will be argued that this diagnostic category provided the clinical precedents and many of the techniques that allowed for congenital word-blindness to become a viable diagnosis. I will describe how acquired word-blindness was used as a point of departure for the crafting of congenital word-blindness. Examining the clinical reasoning connected to the formation of this diagnosis will provide useful insights into the rationalities of government that coalesced to constitute this diagnosis. I will explore how diagnostic categories like acquired word-blindness prepared institutions for categories such as congenital word-blindness to gain institutional acceptance.

My attention shall then turn to the articles that first suggested the possibility of congenital word-blindness. These articles mention their debt to writers studying word-blindness in its acquired form; indeed, Hinshelwood had already established himself as an expert in this area. The emergence of congenital word-blindness from the study of acquired word-blindness will be traced. It shall be suggested that the existence of acquired word-blindness as a legitimate medical diagnosis had established the inability to read or difficulty with reading as a medical concern, albeit with a different aetiology. This constituted the practical conditions and established a vocabulary that made congenital word-blindness a technically feasible diagnosis. The medical concern for a difficulty with reading was, in most cases, a concern with how this difficulty could be overcome. The clinical criteria that were negotiated for congenital word-blindness seem to have been negotiated in relation to rationalities of government concerned with capitalising the population. I will then begin to document how these shifts and alterations were fought over by a variety of experts, and the reasons they gave for their clinical and non-clinical views, convictions and arguments. Debates between medical experts that may initially seem technical, and obscure and clinical in their character can sometimes be re-cast as debates concerning the proper way in which to govern a population.

Aphasias and the Acquiring of a Difficulty with Reading

Johannes Schimdt, a Prussian physician who practised in Danzig during the 1600s, is widely credited with providing the first medical report of a patient who was unable to read for non-optical reasons. The patient that Schimdt discusses had apparently lost the ability to read as a consequence of a severe stroke. Schimdt's case is important as he situates the aetiology of the condition as cerebral rather than optical (Anderson and Meir-Hedde, 2001: 9–10). This move makes reading difficulties a concern within the medical field. A concern, while established, does not disperse beyond this initial site. It does not proliferate around the medical profession.

Schimdt's articles presented his patient as remaining in control of their other intellectual 'faculties'. The loss of the ability to read is positioned as a specific loss of one faculty among many. The loss of the ability to read is distinguished from a variety of intellectual capacitates. Intelligence is here constituted as being made up of several coalescing attributes. This isolation of one intellectual attribute among many will become an important part of the diagnostic criteria in the majority of the articles I discuss in future chapters. Perhaps Schmidt's concern with reading difficulties did not proliferate throughout the medical profession during this period precisely because the necessary technical conditions did not exist. Intelligence, for instance, was not yet understood as being made up of multiple attributes.

After Schmidt, there is relative silence. Nothing is written concerning the loss of the ability to read for more than 200 years. The diagnosis did not take flight. The silence was broken when Sir W.H. Broadbent delivered his paper 'Cerebral Mechanisms of Speech and Thought' to the Royal Medical and Chirurgical Society in 1872. The lack of interest in Schmidt's paper for more than 200 years identifies that although acquiring a difficulty with reading was technically possible within the field of medicine, the conditions for its proliferation as a widely deployed diagnostic category had not yet been established. Broadbent's paper was the first of hundreds, if not thousands, that would be published as the nineteenth century drew to a close and the twentieth century began. The silence concerning reading difficulties ended with an avalanche of reports, articles and case studies.

This book attempts to investigate how this silence was ended. My attention is therefore drawn to many of the earliest articles concerned with word blindness, which allow me to discuss the formation of the diagnosis, its diagnostic criteria and the operations it performed. Several specific questions arise from this work: How was a difficulty with reading re-articulated as a concern of physicians in the period?; How did this question transform into a diagnosis with numerous articles published concerning it when previously it had been ignored? This will be achieved by an attempt to map the solidification and ossification of the diagnosis, so that an examination of how such a diagnosis became an accepted and widely used medical tool at the end of the nineteenth century, even though it had been basically ignored since its introduction in the sixteenth century. This examination asks whether the move towards a bio-politics described in Chapter 2, and a shift in the style of governing reading from one that was concerned with limiting readers to one concerned with proliferating this skill amongst the body of the population, created a hospitable environment for a diagnosis concerned with congenital reading difficulties. In 1825, Bouillaud inaugurated a style of thought that conceived of the loss of cognitive functions, and with it initiated a particular style of writing about the loss of these abilities (Jacyna, 1994: 333). Bouillaud used case studies to describe how patients effectively lost their subjectivity (Jacyna, 1994: 360). This style of writing was dominant in aphasiology during the nineteenth and early twentieth centuries (Jacyna, 2000). This style of writing about aphasia entwines with the rise of the medical profession and its articulation into the activity of government (Osborne, 1993, 1997). This articulation can be seen in the 1870s when, as Rose argues, the medical and psychological professionals moved from a concern with individuals accredited as defective to a concern with defective populations (Rose, 1984: 161).

Broadbent's (1872) 'Cerebral Mechanisms of Speech and Thought' recounted the cases of ten patients with different forms of aphasia. Two of Broadbent's case study patients had lost the ability to read after a brain injury. Broadbent situated these characteristics as aphasic. For the first time since Schmidt, the inability to read or write had come under the auspices of a physician's expertise; medicine was now able to conceptualise and describe a difficulty with reading using its own terminology, vocabulary and concepts. Through a description of these ten cases, Broadbent deployed neurological descriptions to describe why his patients had lost different abilities to differing degrees after various injuries to their brains. Inscribing different intellectual attributes onto different parts of the brain paved the way for a specific diagnosis to be constituted to describe a loss of each of each intellectual attribute due to brain injury.

The first significant terminological shift occurred five years later when Kussmaul introduced the term 'acquired word-blindness'. This diagnosis was used to describe adult patients who were unable to read after experiencing a stroke or injury, and yet were considered to be exhibiting, in all other ways, normal sensory acuity and a 'normal' or better intellect. In other words, their intelligence and sensory acuity had remained, but they had lost the ability to read. Kussmaul (1877) suggested that his patients were experiencing a receptive aphasia. Here, word blindness, while still a type of aphasia, takes the first steps towards becoming a distinct and tangible phenomenon by acquiring its own name. The introduction of a more precise technical terminology, 'acquired word-blindness', is an invention of a diagnostic category somewhat autonomous from aphasia and should be understood as the fashioning of a new instrument—a new technology of power. The development of a precise technology concerned with diagnosing those who had lost the ability to read should be understood as an indication of the problematic identified by Broadbent, taking flight and being crafted into a diagnostic device. Broadbent's insights proliferated where Schmidt's first diagnosis two centuries earlier had not.

In December 1895 a Glaswegian assistant eye surgeon published a paper in *The Lancet* that he had previously read to the Glasgow Medico-Chirurgical Society; the paper was 'Word Blindness and Visual Memory'. The author was James Hinshelwood. It is significant to acknowledge that the paper was delivered by an eye surgeon, as Broadbent had approached the work from the perspective of a general physician. The articulation of the problem by a specialist, in this case an eye specialist, associated the diagnosis with a variety of other specialist technologies. Hinshelwood's paper provides a slightly more precise, more specific aetiology for word-blindness than Kussmaul. Hinshelwood suggests that word-blindness is caused by an injury to the part of the brain concerned with visual memory. Hinshelwood builds upon the work undertaken by Broadbent (1872), where he locates particular intellectual skills in certain regions of the brain. By explaining the loss of a particular attribute upon damage to a specific part of the brain, acquired word-blindness is positioned as a phenomenon engendered by an acquired difference with an individual's brain, specifically the region of the brain concerned with visual memory.

Hinshelwood's (1895) article merits a detailed discussion as within it there is an important review of many English, French and German articles concerned with word-blindness, which had been published in response to the concern with aphasia opened by Broadbent (1872), Kussmaul (1877) and Schmidt. Hinshelwood (1895) does, however, problematise the assertion that all these writers are dealing with the same phenomenon. Hinshelwood asserts that the symptoms and behaviours understood as word-blindness are, in fact, numerous, distinct 'conditions'. As such, he attempts to separate them conceptually and clinically. This is important as it suggests an attempt to refine a diagnostic device, calibrating it to have a more precise function and stamping his mark on the various possible diagnoses:

> It was Kussmaul who first clearly pointed that blindness for words is capable of being met with clinically as an isolated condition and that it represents the pathological condition of a special faculty. He invented the term 'word-blindness' for the condition in which the patient, though not blind, is unable to read visible words. Since Kussmaul's treatise our knowledge of the condition has been greatly increased by the numerous cases which have been reported. It is now evident that the terms 'word-blindness', 'cécité verbale,' and 'Wortblindheit' are not sufficiently precise without further definition. There are different forms of word-blindness which must be carefully distinguished from one another. The case just reported is really one of letter-blindness—i.e., the inability to recognise individual letters. In my case the inability embraced all the different forms of letter know to the patient—Gothic and Latin, written and printed. This is not always so. A few cases have been recorded where the visual memory lost for one alphabet was persevered for another.

Michel quotes a cases where the patient could read the Gothic but not the Latin characters. Charcot had a case where a patient knowing French, German, Spanish, Latin and Greek lost the memory of a few of the Greek and German characters only Mierzejewski has recently described a new of word-blindness which he proposed to call 'caecitas syllabaris et verbalis, sed non litteralis.' The patient could recognise the individuals and name them but he could not unite them into syllables and words. Badal has reported a somewhat similar case which merits more detailed description. (1895: 1565)

Hinshelwood is concerned with the conflation of several different phenomena under the same diagnostic criteria—he is engaged with defining the boundaries of what characteristics can and cannot be considered to be word-blindness. He therefore wishes to distinguish between (1) Kussmaul's conception of word-blindness as the loss of the ability to read words of all language; (2) Charcot's *cécité verbale*, where the patent was accredited with losing the ability to read in several languages and had lost the memory of many characters, but had retained the memory of some German and Greek characters; and (3) Mierzejewski's *caecitas syllabaris et verbalis, sed non litteralis*, where the patient had remembered the names of characters, but was unable to interpret them in blocks as syllables or words. This review of the literature allowed Hinshelwood to engineer his diagnosis so that it performed a more precise function. By refining the function of the diagnosis he was proposing, he distinguished it from related phenomena. This carefully engineered conception of word-blindness allowed Hinshelwood to establish reasons to differentiate between various kinds of aphasia that had hitherto been conflated as the same diagnosis. Calibrating distinct diagnoses for precise characteristics constituted diagnostic categories that, as technologies of power, were able to perform more precise functions than a wider category like aphasia.

Various types of aphasia with similar symptoms were established but crucially differentiated from one another, making the accredited differences more legible at a conceptual, clinical and administrative level. These diagnoses made the characteristics they described more visible. Hinshelwood presented further criticisms of the terminology used to describe these characteristics, focusing on the imprecision of the instruments available:

It is thus evident that the terms 'word-blindness' and 'alexia' are not sufficiently precise. The inability to read may be due to the inability to recognise the individual letters caecitas litteralis, or to an inability to combine these into syllables and words, caecitas syllabaris et verballis. My case affords a remarkably pure example of caecitas litteralis, or inability to recognise the individual letters. (1895: 1566)

Here, Hinshelwood (1895) is stating how, in the case being described, the diagnosis word-blindness, or alexia, is inappropriate. In the case being recounted, it was the memory of individual letters that the patient has lost, rather than words themselves. He thus develops two new terms for the case in question—letter-blindness and *caecitas litteralis*—to more accurately describe the condition he was accrediting his patient as having. The precise calibrating of Hinshelwood's diagnosis illustrated how the government of reading had changed from being purely concerned with how to limit those who had access to this potent art into an attempt to re-imbue the competency to read in those who had lost it. Technical and precise medical diagnoses were being articulated into the government of reading. Like many areas during the late nineteenth and early twentieth centuries (Rose, 1993, 1996a), a variety of technical machinery was being articulated into a specific field as a rationality of acting upon the population as capital was disseminated throughout society.

In the paper 'Word-blindness and Visual Memory' (1895), Hinshelwood proves himself to be capable of innovating precise instruments to describe particular human characteristics and allow for their government. Through analysing numerous cases of 'word-blindness' and related phenomena, re-iterating their key points, Hinshelwood was able to introduce numerous new diagnostic categories—'mind-blindness', 'letter-blindness' and bringing the concept 'Note-blindness' to English readers (Hinshelwood, 1900b). These diagnostic categories operated as new techniques for visualising difference. Building upon the work of Broadbent (1872), intelligence was segmented into various attributes, with a particular aphasia being constituted to describe the loss of one of these attributes. Through using the technical mechanisms produced in Binet's work to diagram the brain, and Broadbent's (1872) work on cerebral mechanisms of speech and thought in order to position the visual memory in a specific region of the brain, Hinshelwood was able to establish how the numerous different varieties of 'word-blindness' and related phenomena may be related to different injuries to the brain. Hinshelwood's conceptual tools were based on his acute knowledge of studies of the brain and its relation to visual memory. His diagnosis worked in assemblage with these technologies when it performed its functions. It is this toolkit that allowed Hinshelwood to give precise cerebral aetiologies for the different varieties of word-blindness, letter blindness, note-blindness and mind-blindness, positioning them in different gryi of an individual's brain.

Hinshelwood makes a brief mention of the possibility of overcoming word-blindness through training or other similar endeavours. This gives an indication of the rationale behind the diagnosis and the operation it serves—to identify patients so they can be subjected to the correct tactics of government:

> of the most interesting features in this case was the slow but gradual improvement of the patient, which I have already described in detail. In most of the recorded cases of word-blindness, unfortunately, there is no account of their after history. In the after histories which are given the patients seem only very rarely to have recovered the power of reading. We know that in aphasia, particularly in youthful patients, the power of speech is sometimes recovered even after complete destruction of the speech centre in the left side of the brain. That the recovery in these cases is due to education of the corresponding centre in the opposite side is, I think, demonstrated by Barlow's case of cerebral lesion, first in the left third frontal convolution and then in the corresponding convolution of the right side. (1895: 1569)

This strategy for helping these patients recover the ability to read, relied upon developing abilities associated with other regions of the brain to compensate for the 'loss' engendered by the injury. This tactic was later utilised as a means of educating and training children diagnosed with congenital word-blindness and remains a method utilised by specialists concerned with educating dyslexic students today. A subject's brain thus came to be seen as a malleable organ that could be cultivated and trained through the deployment of specific and carefully structured practices and procedures. This, of course, fits with the capitalisation of bodies that I have argued characterises bio-politics (see Chapter 2), but with an added dimension. Technologies were being produced to engage in an anatamo-politics of the individual body which acted upon sites that were previously considered ungovernable—particular sections of the human brain. These technologies, like the norm (Ewald, 1990), allowed for the generalisation of power from the individual to the population.

The critique of the imprecise character of the terminology being used is raised again. In the conclusion to this article, Hinshelwood again repeats his discomfort with the term 'blindness' being used in relation to this diagnosis, stating:

> I would ask, why have we such scanty records of cases of mind-blindness, or, as I prefer to designate them, cases of loss of visual memory? I venture to affirm that through lack of knowledge the true nature of such cases, when they do occur, is very frequently not recognized. I would urge the most careful examination of all patients suffering from visual derangements where there are no ocular changes to account for them. It is only by the painstaking analysis of symptoms and the careful recording of such cases, followed, where possible, by pathological examination, that we can hope to gain any further knowledge of the complex cerebral processes involved in vision, of which at present we can only form a very faint and imperfect conception. (1895: 1569–70)

Hinshelwood finds the term 'loss of visual memory' more appropriate than 'mind-blindness'. The accuracy of 'blindness' in describing a particular element of these diagnoses is thus called into question, as the aetiology of the phenomenon being discussed is understood to be cerebral, rather then optical, in its origin. It was necessary to refine the terminology associated with a diagnosis, as part of a general tactic to refine a technology, so that it could articulate relations of power onto specific populations and in an exact fashion. Hinshelwood's anxieties about term 'word-blindness' were shared with other aphasia experts focusing on speech and writing difficulties (such as the 1872 article I discussed earlier and the writers that will be discussed in the following).

As Broadbent was the author of the article that raised reading difficulties within the medical field after a 200 year silence, his intervention is important. Broadbent finds the terminology associated with the diagnosis to be misleading, stating that 'in his judgement the employment of the term word-blindness has been misleading and unfortunate' (in Hinshelwood, 1896: 1453). The debates over terminology that later came to play such an important role in the history of dyslexia (see Chapters 5 and 6) were present before anybody had been diagnosed as having a congenital difficulty with reading.

The term 'mind-blindness' was proclaimed as inaccurate and problematic. Therefore, the 'loss of visual memory' was established as the preferred term. A neurological category was being carved out of a problematic initially raised within the wider medical field. Hinshelwood's hostility to the term blindness was owing to his belief that it inaccurately positions the aetiology of these various aphasias upon the wrong part of the human body, a problem that is accentuated for the conditions of letter- and word-blindness because their diagnosable manifestation happens in relation to printed material. Hinshelwood elaborates on Broadbent's (1872) work and recalibrates acquired word-blindness as a neurological, rather than optical, diagnosis. Examinations were also proposed for all patients suffering from visual derangements where there was no ocular change to account for them. The examination was seen as the primary method of gaining information about the character of word-blindness.

Examinations are to be understood as a technique of the anatamo-politics of the individual body, described by Foucault as emerging before relations of bio-power and, as such, constituted practices that made bio-politics possible. Examinations often operated in assemblage with technologies such as the norm or normality, and have become one of the major methods by which power is generalised from the individual to the body of the population (Ewald, 1990). The whole assemblage of medicine was reacting to various innovations offered by the numerical plotting of individuals (Hacking, 1982, 1990). These included intelligence quota tests, as well as a shift in rationalities of government described in the following chapters. This resulted in previously existing technologies of power being utilised in new ways (Peterson, 1997; Rose, 1985). Medicine's response to these new instruments is comparable to the invention of the microscope, as the deployment made new layers of human difference visible. Attributes could be studied, experimented upon and ultimately altered. Over the course of the nineteenth century the articulation of relations of power became increasingly microscopic in their focus. This allowed for the population to be effectively managed, regulated and cultivated as a state's most valuable resource. An anatamo-politics of the human body, with specific technologies, such as examinations, allowed for medicine to be articulated into the activity of government when politics became bio-politics.

The terminological controversies and debates around the limits of the diagnostic criteria (Hinshelwood, 1895, 1896, 1900a) should be understood as various figures trying to frame the category and make it a more effective diagnosis. These diagnoses performed a precise operation as an instrument for articulating relations of power in a carefully directed way. Traces and residues of the politics of numerous physicians, ophthalmologists, educationalists and parliamentarians were present in the diagnostic category, through the effects they had on the diagnoses being fashioned.

The individuals involved in this debate were actively articulating relations of power as a means of framing the diagnosis so that it would satisfy their own image of it, ensuring it performed the correct operations. Broadbent was one of the first writers to attempt a significant recalibration of the diagnosis by being somewhat critical of the terminology used to describe these attributes. He wrote a critical note in response to one of Hinshelwood's papers which is recalled by Hinshelwood:

> a convenient word for briefly indicating the character of the case. Sir William Broadbent, in a critical note in The Lancet on my paper, has remarked that 'in his judgment the employment of the term word - blindness' has been misleading and unfortunate. (1896: 1453)

Hinshelwood finds some common ground with Broadbent in finding the way the term 'word-blindness' has been deployed by other writers as problematic. He takes issue not with the tool itself, but rather with those who have used it. For Hinshelwood, acquired word-blindness seems a very useful diagnosis that has been deployed in an inappropriate manner. Hinshelwood is calling, therefore, for terminological refinement, which, of course, is part of the careful calibration of a technology of power:

> Now I quite agree with Sir William Broadbent that the word has frequently been used by writers loosely with different meanings attached to it and therefore it has been frequently misleading. The fault, however, lies, not in the word, but, in the fact that those who use it have not always a clear conception of what Kussmaul meant by it. By the term 'word-blindness' is meant a condition in which with normal vision, and therefore seeing the letters and words distinctly, an individual is no longer able to interpret written or printed language. With a clear understanding of this definition there is nothing misleading about the term, which is a most convenient one for describing a group of cases, which, however, includes several different forms. (1896: 1453)

Hinshelwood attempts to strengthen the diagnostic device 'word-blindness' by re-iterating, clarifying and recalibrating Kussmaul's (1877) initial diagnosis. Hinshelwood wants to cut away the dead wood that has made this diagnosis a less effective device and, in clinical terms, a more contestable diagnosis. Importantly, one of Hinshelwood's diagnostic criterions is 'normal vision'. As we know from Ewald (1990), Hacking

(1982, 1990) and Canguilhem (1989) the 'norm' as a tool of measurement, organisation, and way of understanding human bodies and their particular attributes only emerged in the early nineteenth century. I discussed in Chapter 2 how the norm reconfigured life, and how life was considered by strategies of government concerned with acting upon a whole population. In *The Birth of the Clinic*, Foucault established that 'Nineteenth-century medicine, on the other hand, was regulated more in accordance with normality than with health; it formed concepts and prescribed its interventions in relation to a standard of functioning and organic structure' (1989b: 40). For Foucault, medicine had hitherto 'referred, rather to qualities of vigour, suppleness and fluidity, which were lost in illness and which it was the task of medicine to restore' (1989b: 40). Diagnostic categories that were formed during this period, such as word-blindness, were responding to these shifting poles in how bodies were judged. This perhaps offers one of the first reasons why a concern with the difficulty or inability to read was taken up by some physicians, ophthalmologists and, later, psychologists in the late nineteenth and early twentieth centuries with such gusto, rather then in the 1600s when a similar phenomenon had been diagnosed. The fact that medical researchers could now visualise 'normal vision' using instruments of measurement allowed physicians to speculate that the difficulty or inability to read was not necessarily always optical in origin. Vision could be excluded as a cause if the patient's vision was tested to ascertain whether or not it was normal. A new space was opened up for the aetiology of reading difficulties; the newly diagrammed brain could now be used in conjunction with the concept of normality to alert physicians, ophthalmologists and other medical examiners to the fact that the subject in question differed from the norm in some manner. Diagnostic categories, such as word-blindness, necessitated the existence of the technology of normality and its various derivatives. They were only able to operate when they operated in assemblage with these technologies.

In his 1896 article Hinshelwood provides a technical explanation of the aetiology of word-blindness, relying upon the diagrams of the brain to develop his explanation. This furthers the explanation he provided in his 1895 paper. Again, the debt to Broadbent's (1872) work that diagrammed the brain is evident:

Complete word-blindness involving absolute inability to interpret written or printed language (alexia) is due, as was pointed out in my last paper, either to a lesion in the visual memory centre, which occupies the left supramarginal and angular gyrus, or to a lesion which divides completely the fibres connecting this centre with the visual perceptive centres occupying both occipital lobes chiefly in the neighborhood of the cuneus and calcarine fissure. But if the visual memory centre be itself intact and the conductivity of the connecting fibres be only partially impaired there may not be absolute inability to read (alexia), but there may be very great difficulty in interpreting written or printed symbols (dyslexia). (Hinshelwood, 1896: 1452)

This statement is significant as it is the first time the word dyslexia is used to describe reading difficulties in any English-language article. Hinshelwood's distinction here between alexia as an inability to read and dyslexia as a great difficulty in interpreting written or printed symbols is extremely important as it establishes the possibility of dyslexia being a diagnosis of varying degrees. It also makes the diagnostic boundaries for dyslexia much more flexible and porous than its closet relation, alexia. Dyslexia could thus be a potentially more flexible device then alexia. Hinshelwood isolated this one particular symptom—that for dyslexic sufferers 'there may be very great difficulty in interpreting written or printed symbols'—and in so doing established an economy over which dyslexia could articulate relations of power. Dyslexia operated as a sign to identify individuals as having a great difficulty with reading; a sign that suggests relations of power need to be enacted in a particular fashion upon these bodies. The diagnosis is thus a tool for organising, for segregating and training individuals in a carefully directed manner. It is a technology concerned with segmenting the population. Relations of power, concerned with cultivating and training individuals, then act upon this newly segmented population so that they may overcome this difficulty, or at the very least minimise it.

Hinshelwood takes the term dyslexia from Professor Berlin of Stuggart's paper 'Eine Besondere Art der Wortblindheit (Dyslexia)', where six cases that came to Berlin's attention over the course of twenty years are discussed. This text appears to be the first time this term is deployed. Hinshelwood describes why he chooses to adopt the term dyslexia from Berlin and describes how Berlin came to use this term. Hinshelwood also uses the neurological evidence presented by Berlin to ground his version of the diagnosis:

The term 'dyslexia' applied to these cases by Professor Berlin is a convenient one and I have adopted it as describing the prominent symptom in my case. Professor Berlin regards it as a special form of word-blindness, due to an interruption in the conductivity of the connecting fibres of the visual centre in the lower parietal lobe of the left hemisphere. This view has been borne out by postmortem examination. On the whole, Professor Berlin says post-mortem evidence supports the statement that the anatomical seat of the lesion in dyslexia is to be found in the lower parietal lobe of the left hemisphere, which includes the supra-marginal and angular convolutions. Professor Berlin accounts for the phenomena observed by the hypothesis that the interruption of the connecting fibres is only partial, that the capacity for conduction is reduced to a minimum, and that the slight power of conductivity remaining is rapidly exhausted. This seems a plausible and probable explanation of the rapid failure in the patient's power of reading. In the great majority of cases dyslexia has been found to appear as an early and sometimes as the first symptom of grave organic disease of the brain. Even in such cases frequently the dyslexia gradually improved whilst other grave cerebral symptoms subsequently appeared, such as right-sided hemiplegia; a disturbance of sensation on the right side, right lateral homonymous hemianopsia, and sometimes aphasia. All these later cerebral symptoms pointed to a lesion on the left side of the brain within the area between Broca's convolution, the arm and leg motor centres and the visual centres, and such cases frequently went on by a fatal issue. There is another class of cases referred to by Professor Berlin where dyslexia sometimes appears-viz., in chronic alcoholics. In these cases he found that the disturbance gradually passed away when the alcohol was withheld. (1896: 1453)

The post-mortem examination is here operating as part of an assemblage of technologies to map the brain. Placing the aetiology of the diagnosis upon particular regions of the brain that can be identified through a post-mortem examination connects the diagnosis to organic matter. In doing so it makes the characteristics associated with the diagnosis increasingly veritable. The post-mortem examination allows the physician to see what part of the body is defective. Hinshelwood describes precisely the hypothetical aetiology which causes 'dyslexia', offering several different aetiologies that all refer to diseases or damage to particular parts of the brain. Hinshelwood also agrees with Berlin that dyslexia is often found in chronic alcoholics:

The patient's habits, the continuous improvement when alcohol was withheld, and the non-appearance of any further symptoms of

cerebral diseases all combine to confirm the opinion that the dyslexia was of toxic origin due to disturbed nutrition of the cerebral
centres or connecting fibres from excessive indulgence in alcohol.
(1896: 1453)

Dyslexia caused by alcoholism is given a similar neurological aetiology
to word-blindness acquired through a stroke or another brain injury;
it is understood as being caused by damage to the connecting fibres
between the two lateral hemianopsias. Hinshelwood again builds upon
Broadbent's (1872) work where lead poisoning was identified as a possible cause of one of the individual's poor speech. The link to alcoholism
relates to another strategy of government that was invented during the
nineteenth century, namely eugenics. Eugenics pursued the elimination of degeneracy amongst the population and alcoholism was understood by eugenicists as an undesirable characteristic (Hasian, 1996: 31).
The existence of several 'conditions', the aetiology of which focuses
upon one precise part of the brain, allows for writers concerned with
establishing congenital word-blindness to use the existence of various
acquired forms of word-blindness to increase the validity of their own
research.

Knowledge of the brain gained from post-mortem examinations of
patients, who had experienced either difficulties or the inability to
read, had allowed Hinshelwood and others to produce a diagnosis that
operated from these newly constructed diagrams. An organically veri-
fied diagram of a cerebral difference makes the condition more visible. This diagram of the aetiology of acquired word-blindness focused
upon the connecting fibres between two hemispheres in the brain. It
allowed other reasons for why certain individuals acquired a difficulty
with reading (e.g. alcoholism or lead poisoning) to be included under
the auspices of the diagnosis. An individual who had acquired word-
blindness was understood as having a different cerebral make up to a
'normal' person. This accredited alteration was considered to be due
to an accident or chemical abuse. The diagrams being mapped at this
time for various acquired conditions developed the possibility of similar phenomena existing in a congenital form. Once it had been ascertained that an injury or stroke could affect particular parts of the brain,
and it had been conceived of that these differences caused some individuals to have difficulties with reading, visual memory or organising
information, then it would be hypothesised by the examination that
an individual may have acquired this condition if he/she had difficulty
with these skills. Individuals who were accredited as having normal

brains and then acquired word-blindness, through alcoholism or injury, provided evidence of a possible cerebral difference from which a congenital diagnosis could be formed. The diagnosis of acquired word-blindness made the discipline of medicine hospitable to the possibility of a congenital diagnosis.

A New Diagnosis: Congenital Word-blindness

It was the study of acquired word-blindness which led to the recognition of the cause of the inability or difficulty in learning to read, which is seen in many children, as being due to a congenital defect in the visual memory for words and letters, and which hence could be conveniently described as congenital word-blindness. That these cases are comparatively numerous is now evident from their appearance in large number of ophthalmological journals during the last few years. (Hinshelwood, 1912: 1034)

From the standpoint of the present, the diagnostic categories of congenital word-blindness and alexia describe vastly different phenomena, the former being a relatively common learning difficulty and the latter an uncommon phenomenon associated with brain injuries or a stroke. Yet, at the turn of the nineteenth century, these were diagnoses that were conceived of as being close relations. As Hinshelwood (1912) states, he was led to the study of congenital word-blindness by his earlier work on acquired word-blindness. So, for Hinshelwood, it was the study of acquired word-blindness (and Morgan's 1896 paper) that brought the possibility of congenital word-blindness to his immediate attention. Numerous patients must have had the characteristics later credited as congenital word-blindness, but now medical technologies were able to see them. What had changed? Had the technical instruments of government and the rationality of governing changed to such an extent that reading difficulties were a problem that government should attend to? The reconfiguring of the population engendered by the numerical plotting of bodies and the diagramming of this population in relation to the poles of normality and abnormality had changed how intelligence was conceived and acted upon (see Chapter 2).

These technical and logical changes in the practices of government allowed the problem of reading difficulties to take flight in the nineteenth century. The conditions for it to proliferate were not yet established in the seventeenth century, when it had initially been posited by Schmidt. Relations of power were articulated into technologies concerned with examining, managing and cultivating bodies, thereby augmenting the reach of strategies of government concerned with capitalising the population. Diagnoses hitherto unimaginable became viable objects of study, and offered useful possibilities in the government of the population. The description of how congenital word-blindness relied upon various technological foundations found in the already existing diagnosis of acquired word-blindness could then be conducted. This allowed the diagnosis to achieve a veritable status at a relatively quick pace, as all that was required was for an already expected diagnosis to be recalibrated to fit a new population.

It was not until 1896 that Dr Pringle Morgan reported a case where a patient exhibited a difficulty with reading attributed to a congenital defect. Morgan dubbed this diagnosis congenital word-blindness. Unlike acquired word-blindness, congenital word-blindness was understood to be a form of word-blindness where the characteristics were present within individuals since birth and were not caused by a brain injury. As Morgan states:

> Cases of word blindness are always interesting, and this case is, I think particularly so. It is unique, so far as I know, in that it follows upon no injury or illness, but is evidently congenital, and due most probably to defective development of that region of the brain disease which in adults produces practically the same symptoms—that is, the left angular gryus. (1896: 1378)

Morgan's suggestion of a congenital diagnosis should be considered an epistemological break (Bachelard, 1984). Morgan here makes an extremely important decision in suggesting that this case of word-blindness is due to a developmental difference in the left angular gyrus of the brain. This is an analogous aetiology to that provided in Hinshelwood's (1895) description of acquired word-blindness and also Broadbent's (1872) description of the loss of the ability to read due to brain injury. Morgan's new diagnosis is produced by simply inserting a new prefix and aetiology. It was a fairly simple modification to the technology acquired word-blindness, as the newly formed technology congenital word-blindness relied upon much of the same diagnostic logic. Nonetheless, it was a crucial move as it allowed the diagnostic machinery to be recalibrated to operate upon a new population.

The positioning of the aetiology of congenital word-blindness in a particular region of the brain is a very important development as it makes the characteristics that 'congenital word-blindness' is concerned with visible. By being made visible, I mean that relations of power had coalesced, problematising the characteristics that the diagnosis dealt with. Through this process these characteristics became increasingly visible to experts. The visibility of congenital word-blindness relied upon the work conducted to diagram the brain by Broadbent (1872), where the aetiology was initially established for aphasics who had lost their ability speak or, in two cases, the ability to read. In putting these diagrams to use relations of power were articulated to produce diagnostic categories to describe differences that were previously invisible to the technical tools that medical science had available. This use of Broadbent's diagrams was of particular importance given that he was a physician wielding strong influence within the medical profession, thus giving his research considerable weight.

These differences effectively did not exist until technological advancements and relations of power interacted to make them visible, measurable and, of course, governable. Congenital reading difficulties were made into a possible diagnostic problematic by the coalescing of several technologies of power and rationalities of government. This marked a shift in how reading was governed, in the development of various methods of numerically plotting the population, in the development of technologies to assess and measure individual attributes, and signalled a general shift towards a style of government that was bio-political in its character. Congenital word-blindness was given a physical aetiology, even though it was invisible to the naked eye. It is important to note that Morgan's (1896) proposition of the diagnosis congenital word-blindness refers directly to the literature on acquired word-blindness, building on its assumptions and using its technological components to constitute a diagnosis that acts upon a new population. The closeness of the diagnosis' aetiology to an already existing condition increases its visibility, and also its believability, by making links to an established diagnostic category. From its initial announcement in the pages of *The Lancet*, Morgan was able to utilise the capillaries of power that had already been established by research concerned with acquired word-blindness as a means of giving his newly proposed diagnosis a clinical foundation. Hinshelwood had proposed that dyslexia was a 'severe', acquired 'difficulty' with reading (1896: 1453). Reading difficulties were therefore already an established problem that medicine had a jurisdiction over, and congenital word-blindness could be formed by a subtle alteration to an already existing technology. It was essentially produced by recalibrating already existing machinery and replacing a single component: its aetiology. This newly constituted diagnostic machinery allowed for the recognition of a new population, and for relations of power to act upon this population. The flow of power onto a completely different set of bodies required only the smallest recalibration of an already existing technology.

The medical examination of patients had been the primary method of diagnosing individuals as having acquired word-blindness. This technique was also utilised in data gathering and diagnosing congenital word-blindness. Morgan describes the case of a fourteen-year-old boy who appeared to have developed 'normally'—a category, a technology, that will prove absolutely essential to those who formed the diagnosis congenital word-blindness:

> He has always been a bright and intelligent boy, quick at games, and in no way inferior to others in his age. His great difficulty has been, and is now his inability to learn to read. This inability is so remarkable, and so pronounced, that I have no doubt it is due to some congenital defect. (1896: 1378)

Morgan goes to great lengths to disqualify the possibility that the boy he is writing about should not be understood as 'feeble-minded'. It thus becomes important to establish that he is 'bright', 'intelligent', 'quick at games' and, most importantly, 'no way inferior to others in his age'—the boy is thus presented to us as being 'normal', or even above average. It is made clear that the boy's only difficulty—the only way he differs from other 'normal' children—is in regard to his inability to read. The diagnosis requires the technology of normality to make the assessment. It is important to note that the first cases of congenital word-blindness are where the subject is accredited as being unable to read, which is different from a difficulty with reading. It is recounted that this inability is so 'remarkable and so pronounced' that Morgan can have no doubt in asserting, in the case of this boy, that there is a 'congenital defect', which causes his inability to read. Morgan thus presents a great chasm between the boy's general intelligence and his inability to read. It is the degree of this great difference that makes the case interesting for medicine. The patient's status as being in all other ways 'normal' or 'above average' thus marks him as a subject worthy of being cultivated. Again, the technology of the norm is being used to measure the patient. In this case it is used to evaluate whether the localised nature of the difficulty marks the subject as being worthy of further attention. Congenital word-blindness and the norm are being deployed as an assemblage operating upon the body to articulate relations of power in an anatamo-politics of the human body. As Ewald (1991) has suggested the norm articulated relations of power in a disciplinary way allowing power to be generalised from an anatamo-politics of the human body to a bio-politics of the population. Congenital word-blindness also operated as a sign that allowed for the better management of people with varying degrees of intelligence—individuals who, apart from their difficulty with reading, were otherwise accredited as being very bright could now be understood as being different from individuals considered to have a more general 'lack of intelligence'.

The localised character of the characteristics accredited as a defect allowed for the precise micro-management of educational attributes by identifying those who had a localised congenital difficulty with reading. The invention of this diagnosis through the recalibration of already existing diagnostic machinery fits within a general move with medical science, wherein technologies of power were operating on increasingly specific populations: segmenting, classifying and re-ordering bodies (Osborne, 1993, 1997; Rose, 1984, 1999). These technical developments allowed medicine to articulate relations of power in an increasingly microscopic fashion. Examining bodies was critical to the possibility of creating such a diagnostic machinery. The anatamo-politics of the human body thus facilitated the formation of the bio-politics of the population. The examination thus provided information to those concerned with the government of children. This knowledge fabricated a new economy through which power could operate—children, and their potential skills, were now an object that could be managed, developed and cultivated through particular kinds of intervention. By sifting out from those accredited as feeble-minded a different and distinct population—those whose difficulties were localised could be obtained. Crucially, the localised character of these difficulties meant they could be overcome.

Robert Castels (1991) has illustrated how a change in the government of dangerous individuals occurred during the nineteenth century, as the emphasis shifted from the use of confinement and reactive medical techniques to attempts to govern the risk of undesirable events such as deviant behaviour or illness. In this sense, medicine should be understood as being articulated into the activity of governing 'risky individuals'. Governing risky individuals is made possible by the numerical plotting of the population (discussed in Chapter 2). This style of government actually eschews the government of individuals and focuses instead on populations, as by using 'statistical correlations of heterogeneous elements, the experts have multiplied the possibilities for preventive intervention' (Petersen, 1997: 193). By being articulated into the government of risk, medicine begins to operate according to the logic of a governmentality that is concerned with the future rather than the present.

Following Thomas Osborne, I would argue that medicine gets articulated into the activity of statecraft by becoming concerned with cultivating the value of the population. As the medical professional is articulated into the activity of government '[i]t is as if the territory and occupants of the state have taken on a kind of autonomous value' (1997: 176). The health, abilities and attributes of a population therefore gain value, and at the same time form a greater focus on distinguishing between different elements of the population accredited as being feeble-minded, backward or defective. A search begins for what bodies could overcome localised difficulties. This should be understood as a response to medicine being articulated into the activity of government, now having at its disposal increasingly microscopic techniques resulting from the numerical plotting of the population.

Morgan recounts the case of a boy who has attended school or been in some other form of education since the age of seven, and that continual and great efforts have been made to teach the boy to read. However, 'in spite of this laborious and persistent training, he can only with difficulty spell out words of one syllable' (1896: 1378). The 'normality' of the boy is continually proclaimed throughout the article. It is continually suggested that the boy is in no way inferior to his peers. The boy, however, is said to have difficulty with the lexicon, finding reading and writing both formidable tasks. Morgan attempts to present the boy's difficulty with the lexicon as being peculiar in the context of the rest of his intelligence by illustrating the boy's excellent ability with mathematical problems and his ability to read numerical figures. This establishes his difficulties with reading as being a localised problem in an otherwise intelligent individual. The argument that is presented is that, despite the boy's otherwise 'normal' intelligence, his difficulties with reading and writing have hampered his performance in education. By proclaiming the boy as being 'normal' in other ways, apart from his difficulty with reading, this phenomenon is isolated. Its isolation means that it can be concentrated upon by specialists. This microscopic element of a patient's intelligence can now be acted upon with precision in the hope of overcoming, or at least minimising, this boy's accredited defective attribute so that he might pass as normal. If, as I have argued, bio-politics is characterised, in part, by the development of a rationale whereby the body of the population came to be understood as capital, then congenital word-blindness operated as a technology that tried to filter a group of bodies from the category of the feeble-minded that perhaps could be cultivated.

The boy described by Morgan was being problematised. This problematisation did not occur in a single site—the school, home or the clinic. It occurred in all of these and, no doubt, in others, as the logic of seeing bodies as capital was diffusing throughout society (Foucault, 1977, 2003). The introduction of mass education by the Elementary Education Act of 1870 meant that boys, such as the one described by Morgan, had to be schooled. As mainstream education did not benefit this boy—the boy did not respond to the articulation of various technologies of power and therefore he was identified as being different; his difference was problematised. It was the possibility of localising his difficulty to a particular set of intellectual attributes that differentiated him from those accredited as being feeble-minded. His schoolmaster recollected that the boy would have been the smartest boy in school if instruction were entirely oral. The educational system thus relied upon medical authority to legitimise this difference and to find ways of identifying children who had problems with specific areas of the curriculum that hampered their education. The machineries of education and medicine were operating in assemblage with one another.

The research into congenital word-blindness and similar formations was orientated towards the identification, measurement and management of educational difference. Medical professionals were thus articulated into the activity of education by producing diagnoses that segmented the educational population based on particular intellectual attributes. Society was not being medicalised. Rather, the technologies of medicine were now more useful and freely available to administrators of various kinds. Medicine, like so many other institutions and disciplines during the period, was being articulated into the activity of government.[1] Medicine could now be deployed to provide expertise and evidence in the process of the cultivation of bodies who were otherwise codified as normal (despite their reading difficulty) into productive and skilled bodies. The invention of congenital word-blindness should be understood as the fashioning of a specific technology in response to this shift in practices of government. The articulation of ophthalmology into the activity of governing educational difference should be understood as part of the articulation of the professions, particularly the medical profession, into the activity of statecraft (Osborne, 1997: 176).

Morgan's paper was followed in 1900 by Hinshelwood's 'Congenital Word-blindness'. Hinshelwood took up the subject of writing about congenital word-blindness with gusto, publishing several articles and reports on the patients he diagnosed (1900a, 1990b, 1904, 1907). It, of course, makes sense that an expert who already had significant knowledge of the diagnosis would take a leading part in the recalibration of the technological machinery so that a new diagnostic device could be invented. Writing on reading difficulties gave Hinshelwood the opportunity to branch out of optical concerns into neurology. Technological innovations were deployed and were used in assemblage to re-imagine and constitute a specific population. They were ultimately made visible by the numerical plotting of the individual mind that was carried out in scientific studies of the brain and mind, and by allowing for a comparison between bodies within a population. The numerical plotting of individuals and populations appears to have been a necessary condition for congenital word-blindness to operate. This plotting of the brain constituted a machinery of government that worked in assemblage with technologies of power, such as the norm (Ewald, 1990), allowing for an anatamo-politics of the human body to be generalised into a bio-politics of the population. It allowed for differences in individual cerebral characteristics to be measured and recorded in a standardised manner, thus making possible the identification of populations who shared similar characteristics. The rise of professions, and the increasing articulation of medicine and its allied sciences into the activity of government made individual bodies increasingly calculable (Miller, 1992).

The importance of neurology was in grounding the diagnosis in a veritable diagram and allowing for the characteristics that congenital word-blindness represented to be mapped onto this diagram. Hinshelwood's description of the cerebral process of reading deploys many neurological concepts and is similar to the descriptions found in Broadbent (1872):

> With this understanding of the processes involved in acquiring the art of reading by sight our cases became quite clear and intelligible. The difficulty experienced by these patients in learning to read arose from the fact that their visual memory for words and letters was congenitally defective. I have shown in my former papers that there is a definite cerebral area within which these visual memories of words and letters are registered-viz., the angular supra-marginal gyrus on the left side of the brain in right-handed people. If there be any abnormality within this area, due either to disease, to injury at birth, or to defective development, it is easily conceivable how such an individual should experience great difficulty in learning to read.

The degree of difficulty may vary greatly in different cases. (1896: 1507)

Hinshelwood draws upon his previous research into acquired word-blindness, where he established a definite cerebral area within which the memories of words and letters are registered—the supra-marginal gyrus on the left of the brain of right-handed individuals—to provide a neurologically-based aetiology of congenital word-blindness. Hinshelwood is thus establishing capillaries between the two diagnoses, using the work he and others had already conducted to give the diagnosis respectability and grounding. Through utilising his previous research, it is evident that Hinshelwood was recalibrating a previously established technology in order for it to perform an alternative operation on a distinct population. In Hinshelwood's (1895) previous work he suggested that the part of the brain that dealt with visual memory was the supra-marginal gyrus on the left of the brain of right-handed people. The description Hinshelwood gives of the boy earlier in his paper emphasises how, through measuring his auditory memory and visual memory, the boy is identified as having a significant discrepancy between the two:

CASE 1.-A boy, aged 11 years, was at school for four and a half years, but was finally sent away because he could not be taught to read. His father informed me that he was a considerable time at school before the defect was noted, as he had such an excellent memory that he learned his lessons by heart; in fact, his first little reading-book he knew by heart, so that whenever it came to his turn he could from memory repeat his lesson, although he could not read the words. His father also informed me that in every respect, less his inability to learn to read the boy seemed quite as intelligent as any of his brothers and sisters. His auditory memory was excellent and better than that of any of the other members of the family. When a passage was repeated to him aloud he could commit it to memory very rapidly. When I first saw the boy and his father at the Glasgow Eye Infirmary I asked them to call on me at my house, and I wrote down the address on an envelope. A few days thereafter the father could not find the envelope, but the boy at once repeated the address correctly, having remembered it from hearing me state it once. I examined the boy first on March 4th, 1900, when he seemed a smart and intelligent lad for his years. He knew the alphabet by heart, repeating it rapidly and correctly. He could recognise by sight, however, only a very few letters and those not with any degree of certainty. He could spell correctly most simple words of one syllable such as 'cat,' 'dog,' 'man,' 'boy,' &c., but he could not recognise by sight the simplest and commonest words, such as 'the,' 'of,' 'in,' 'to' &c. He had no difficulty in recognising all other visual objects, such as faces, places, and pictures. (1900a: 1506)

According to Hinshelwood's description, the father seems adamant in emphasising the boy's intelligence despite his difficulty with reading. This father had obviously recognised the importance of establishing that his child was intelligent despite his localised difficulty with reading. The desire to distinguish this boy from the population accredited as feeble-minded emanated from his father, as well as his schoolteachers. Hinshelwood reproduces the information that the boy's father gave him. The necessity to make the distinction clear between a boy like the one being discussed and a child classified as feeble-minded is established. The exceptional feats of the boy's memory are presented to make it clear to the reader that this boy should be treated differently to those accredited as feeble-minded. Information about the boy's ability to remember visual objects provides further credence to the claim that there is a part of the brain concerned with interpreting and remembering symbols. The description makes clear that the boy's difficulty is isolated, and, in fact, in all other ways he is exceptionally intelligent. Hinshelwood describes the precise character of the boy's difficulty with his lexicon:

Although he had not been able to learn to recognise by sight the letter and words in his little primer he could repeat the content of the book by heart. He could repeat the alphabet correctly and rapidly, but he could only recognise some of the letters by sight and then often after many mistakes. He could spell rapidly and correctly most words of one syllable such as 'cat,' 'dog,' 'boy,' 'man,' &c., but he could not recognise by sight one of these words. Even such common words as 'the,' 'of,' 'in,' 'to,' &c., he could not recognise by sight although he could spell them quite correctly. The failure of visual memory was for words and letters only. It did not extend to objects, persons, places. Pictures of all kinds he recognised at once. It was therefore perfectly clear that the difficulty lay in the failure of the visual memory for letters and words. In this lad's case the defect was extreme, as even after years of practice he had not been able to acquire visual memories of all the letters of the alphabet. (1896: 1508)

Hinshelwood then goes on to explain a phenomenon he had already encountered in some of his earlier papers, namely that individuals with acquired word or letter blindness can sometimes still read and interpret figures:

> It is there argued that the complete functional independence of the visual memories of letters, words, and numbers, as evidenced by the fact that many patients completely word- and letter-blind can still read figures, could only be satisfactorily explained by anatomical independence-i.e., that these memories were registered in different areas of the cerebral cortex. From this point of view it is easily understood how these four patients, while experiencing the very greatest difficulty in learning to read letters and words, had little or none in learning to read figures. (1896: 1508)

Hinshelwood's solution is to suggest that different parts of the brain are concerned with interpreting words and letters rather than figures, and that 'defects' in the parts of the brain concerned with interpreting 'symbols', 'figures', or 'musical notes' will engender the characteristics that, in regard to reading, are referred to as congenitally word-blind. Again, this follows on from Broadbent's (1872) paper. The attributing of different intellectual attributes onto two different parts of the brain allows for the segmenting of the population based upon a localised congenital difficulty with one of these attributes.

Owing to the small number of cases reported at this point it would, perhaps, have been safe to assume that the case was rare. However, the rarity of this condition is called into question by Hinshelwood:

> Although I have not been able to bring forward more than these four cases as illustrations of this congenital form of 'Word-blindness' I have but little doubt that these are by no means so rare as the absence of recorded cases would lead us to infer. Their rarity is, I think, accounted for by the fact that when they do occur they are not recognised. It is a matter of the highest importance to recognise the cause and the true nature of this difficulty in learning to read which is experienced by these children, otherwise they may be harshly treated as imbeciles or incorrigibles and either neglected or flogged for a defect for which they are in no way responsible. The recognition of the true character of the difficulty will lead the parents and teachers of these children to deal with them in the proper way, not by harsh and severe treatment, but by attempt-

ing to overcome the difficulty by patient and persistent training. (1896: 1508)

Although the cases of word-blindness seem to have just appeared on the medical professional's field of perception, Hinshelwood still rallies against the argument that this condition is rare, instead asserting that these children may have been previously 'unfairly' understood as 'imbeciles or incorrigibles'. This paves the way for the diagnosis to be articulated onto a wider population. Children accredited as having congenital word-blindness are once again distinguished from those accredited as being 'feeble-minded' (research into the 'feeble-minded' was a dominant concern of psychology at this point, as has been shown by Rose (1984)). Their common and identifying characteristics are being asserted in an attempt to concretise their separation and differentiation from this group.

Apart from raising the question of what sort of defect a child could be responsible for, the above quotation bears a resemblance to the proclamations made a few decades earlier regarding the deserving poor. Congenital word-blindness is thus presented as a deserving defect (Davis, 1995). Rather than treating these children harshly, Hinshelwood proposes that patient and persistent training methods must be established to help them 'overcome' their difficulty. The character of the boy as deserving is formulated in two ways. First, by a process of differentiation through which the deserving are distinguished from those accredited as feebleminded; and, second, by establishing that they are not in any way responsible for their condition. Those accredited as being feeble-minded could not be cultivated because they were considered to have inferior potential to the rest of the population; their bodies were therefore not amenable to the touch of the technologies of management. Congenital word-blindness opens the possibility of finding members within the feeble-minded population whose difficulties are localised, and who can therefore be cultivated through emphasis on their other attributes. Hinshelwood's argument—that congenital word-blindness is more common than has hitherto been presumed—is therefore a rallying cry to look at the population accredited as feeble-minded and find ways to capitalise it. Congenital word-blindness was a technology precisely calibrated to cultivate value in a resource hitherto thought of as without value. Congenital word-blindness was able to perform the function of taking a population accredited as 'imbeciles or incorrigibles' and identifying that a proportion of this population had the potential to be governed differently because, if the correct techniques were applied, they would be able to benefit from education.

Conclusion

This chapter has described how a particular set of characteristics became problematised by the new concern of medical professionals in the late nineteenth century. An outline has been provided of how reading difficulties were re-established as a medical concern after first being proposed in the 1600s. The first reading difficulties to be diagnosed in the nineteenth century were aphasic conditions. Acquired reading difficulties were diagnosed before congenital ones, as medicine's concern was initially with defective individuals rather than defective populations. Compulsory education had only been in place for a matter of years when Broadbent (1872) and Kusmaul (1877) wrote of cases of acquired word-blindness. Children with the characteristics that would later become understood as congenital word-blindness were not yet problematised as they didn't have to attend school.

I have argued that acquired word-blindness provided a diagram, albeit one connected to organic evidence, that allowed for congenital reading difficulties to be invented as a diagnosis. The diagnosis was made possible by a medical gaze resulting from the formation of a diagram of human characteristics and capabilities that departed from the restrictions of the five human senses. The eyes of those concerned with governing relied less on human vision and increasingly on the sight of technical instruments. The careful recalibration of the aetiology of the diagnosis—'acquired word-blindness'—allowed for congenital word-blindness to operate upon a new population. The process of the formation of the diagnosis congenital word-blindness is therefore related to the development of aphasic diagnostic categories. When this new diagnosis, 'congenital word-blindness', was formed and diagnosed in 1895, it performed the operation of distinguishing between what bodies in the population accredited as feeble-minded could, in fact, be cultivated. This strategy of capitalising the population is related to the rise of the professions, particularly medical professions. It is also related to the formation of eugenic and socially hygienic ways of thinking about the population that saw the population as a resource. These factors coalesced to make it problematic if an individual body was not equipped with the skills they were expected to be in possession of (Hasian, 1996: 35).

Reading had become an obligatory requirement, as the economy was increasingly reliant upon literate bodies. Finding ways to increase the value of a resource was part of the logic of capitalism, a logic now applied to both the bodies. Congenital word-blindness was a technology concerned with fostering value in sites that had previously been considered to be valueless; in this case, finding a cultivatable subgroup from within the population accredited as feeble-minded. Congenital word-blindness was fashioned owing to the coalescing of a variety of strategies of government and historical events. The invention of such technologies of power is not surprising as the activity of government had now become concerned with fostering life (Foucault, 1979: 138–43, 2003: 253–63; Hacking, 1982: 281; Rose and Miller, 1992: 174). The liberal style of government depended upon the wide dispersion of expertise (Rose, 1993: 291). The rise of professions converted the multitude into a population of calculable individuals (Miller, 1992). Bio-politics was able to foster worth not only at the level of the population but also on the individual body owing to the formation of numerous experts. The formation of congenital word-blindness can be understood as produced by ophthalmological experts owing to the increased function of professionals within society, which was part of a bio-politics concerned with augmenting value in the population, and triply formed the medical condition of congenital word-blindness. This produced a diagnosis in response to both the now increased function of the professionals and a bio-politics concerned with augmenting value in the population. The articulation of ophthalmology into the activity of governing educational difference should be understood as part of the articulation of the professions, particularly the medical profession, into the activity of statecraft (Osborne, 1997: 176). Hinshelwood's initial version of the diagnosis, as detailed here, described characteristics that, if individuals were found to possess them, then in his opinion they deserved to be given specialist education. The logic that the practices of ophthalmologists followed separated those children who had an isolated difficulty with reading from the population accredited as feeble-minded. Further study of its operation must now be undertaken.

5

The Technological Operation of Congenital Word-blindness: Marking Some Differences as More Deserving Than Others

In the previous chapter the formation of reading difficulties as a medical problem was described. This process lead to the development of two diagnoses: acquired word-blindness as a type of aphasia and congenital word-blindness. I described how the production of congenital word-blindness as a medical condition utilised the technical innovations of acquired word-blindness. As a technology of power, congenital word-blindness was essentially a recalibration of acquired word-blindness. This recalibration allowed for relations of power to be articulated onto a new array of bodies. The scrutiny of my description now moves away from the formation of a precise field of knowledge—the diagnostic category congenital word-blindness—towards a further exploration of how the diagnosis operates as a technology of power. This is a problem that I began to discuss in Chapter 4, and in this chapter I will describe how the diagnosis operates as a specific technology of power, the flow of power to new sites that engender new ways for it to disperse onto bodies and the particular way it then acts upon those bodies. The following discussion is concerned with providing a detailed description of how congenital word-blindness functioned and how its operation was framed by being understood as a problem under the jurisdiction of ophthalmology.

This discussion of the functionality of the diagnosis is split into seven sections. The first is concerned with how the diagnosis operated to differentiate those accredited as congenitally word-blind from both the *normal* and the *abnormal*. The second considers how moral values were attached to the bodies of those being diagnosed and the process of diagnosis itself, and how this imbuing of moral attributes furthered the process of differentiation. The third section details why an early diagnosis was advocated by the ophthalmic writers. This recalls the work on aphasia and looks forward to the future discussion of education. The fourth details how the character of the diagnosis allowed it to function within a pedagogic context, documenting the establishment of links with educational groups. The fifth section describes how the insertion of a hereditary component into the diagnostic machinery altered how it functioned on a specific technical level, and how this transformed the function that the technology could perform when articulated by wider rationalities into the activity of government. The sixth section considers how challenges presented by Claiborne, Jackson and Rutherford (from the USA) offered different political rationalities for diagnosis, with a particular focus on Rutherford's work owing to the distinctiveness of his political programme. The seventh section describes how Hinshelwood responded to deployments of his diagnosis that he did not approve of, and the various criticisms he was presented with.

Numerous papers concerned with congenital word-blindness were published during the period of 1901–09 (Ball, 1907; Bruner, 1905; Claiborne, 1906; Fisher, 1905; Hinshelwood, 1902, 1904, 1907; Jackson, 1906; Nettleship, 1901; Rutherford, 1909; Stephenson, 1907; Thomas, 1905). These will be analysed in this chapter; however, the following discussion will focus predominately upon papers that I consider to represent advances in the diagnostic criteria or which are considered to provide indicative examples of a particular rationality of government. It is striking that the majority of the articles were published in specialist ophthalmology (Hinshelwood, 1902, 1904; Nettleship, 1901) or wider-interest medical journals (Claiborne, 1906; Hinshelwood, 1907; Jackson 1906). The frequent publishing in specialist ophthalmological journals suggests that word-blindness fell under the auspice of ophthalmology. The publication in wider-interest medical journals seems to be a result of the necessity of informing the wider medical community of a significant development in the diagnosis, like the insertion of the hereditary hypothesis (Hinshelwood, 1907; Thomas, 1905), or, indeed, as Hinshelwood and Morgan had done when they were initially introducing the diagnosis to the medical community (Hinshelwood, 1896, 1900a; Morgan, 1896). Claiborne (1906) and Jackson's (1906) papers both present diagnostic and terminological challenges. Both writers were American and performed the task of introducing the diagnosis to a North American audience so as to establish themselves as authorities on the subject.

Congenital word-blindness during the period 1901–09 is an ophthalmological problem. Rutherford's (1909) contribution is one the first examples of word-blindness being considered in a specialist, but nonophthalmological, periodical, as his article was published in the *Journal of Children's Diseases*. The other exception is Lightner Witmer's (1907b) article, which was published in a psychology journal. Strictly speaking, it does not deal with congenital word-blindness, but is later used as a reference point for writers attempting to move the diagnosis under the auspice of psychology. In the interest of thematic continuity, a discussion of this paper has been left for Chapter 6. In the early part of the twentieth century, congenital word-blindness was an ophthalmic problem. In this chapter I will explore why this was the case.

The insertion of the hereditary hypothesis into the diagnosis by Thomas (1905), and the strong institution of a relationship with particular educational machineries, can be analysed as allowing the diagnosis to operate in assemblage with a variety of different technologies of power and machineries of government. The shift in how diagnosis was able to function can be seen in the work of Thomas (1905); Hinshelwood (1907) began to deploy the heredity hypothesis. I will also describe how a distinct shift in the rationalities of government which the diagnosis would be associated with occurred owing to the insertion of this diagnostic component. North American challenges to Hinshelwood are described, as they offered distinct terminological propositions, and seemed to make the diagnosis admissible to political programmes different to those associated with it in the UK. Rutherford's contribution is given significant consideration owing to its radically different conception of the individuals being diagnosed and the distinct operation it performed.

A Technology of Differentiation

A medical diagnosis is a taxonomic device, a technology of power that categorises, organises and manages bodies. Like Bowker and Star (1999: 319) I consider classifications as specific technologies that are inserted into wider infrastructures; technologies of power assembled into a machinery of government that are then articulated by strategies of government. The process of diagnosis allows the medical practitioner to assess what category best describes the individuals' symptoms, behaviour or biological difference. Through this process of assessment and subsequent categorisation, decisions can be made about the appropriate actions to be undertaken (including, of course, the lack of action). The assessor is able to refer treatments or actions considered to be appropriate for the categorisation that has been identified. The ability to diagnose an individual into a particular category is thus essential for recommending what actions the patients should take upon themselves or how others should act upon them. Diagnosing, sorting and categorising allow the activity of government to take place through heterogeneous actions on a diverse array of bodies.

As was discussed in Chapters 2 and 3, the transition from politics to bio-politics reformed many seemingly disparate spaces. The eugenics movement and social hygienism provided two rationalities of government that directed bio-politics onto newly imagined trajectories. Both had been key influences on the formation of the psychology of the individual and had engendered shifts in medical practice in general (Rose, 1984). As Foucault's research has shown (1979, 2003, 2007, 2008), the population had been transformed into a resource—a resource that was at risk of degenerating. The population was now conceived as having the potential to be improved. For Foucault, this way of governing populations was made possible by the new forms of knowledge and, in turn, this style of government exacerbated the need for further expertise of this type. The invention of various psychological tests, and, in particular, intelligence and personality tests, constituted several levels of differentiation that were previously invisible. Eugenic thinking was not a marginal discourse and the effect of its rationalities must not be downplayed when considering the formation or relative solidification of a diagnosis during the period (Hasian, 1996: 30). However, eugenic thinking was not the only rationale concerned with bodies; all politics became bio-politics during the nineteenth century. The mainstream character of eugenic thinking late nineteenth- and early twentieth-century Britain resulted in the eugenic rationale having an influence upon all areas of bio-politics (Hasian, 1996: 35–6).

The norm was not yet a century old (Davis, 1995; Hacking, 1990), yet it had already shown itself to be of great utility. It had achieved significant moral and political currency for a variety of different rationalities of government, potentialities that had only been exacerbated by the eugenics movement. To not be normal was, in many cases, a moral failing of the individual (Bauman, 1991: 32; Davis, 1995: 23–49). It became desirable that the bodies attained certain normal attributes or qualities, as the activity of government became concerned with cultivating certain attributes onto the body of the individual and across the body of the population (Foucault, 1979, 2003, 2007, 2008). The categories of normal and abnormal had great political currency, which was exacerbated by their recently discovered utility in psychology and education (Rose, 1985, 1999). It was between these two poles that the emergent diagnosis of congenital word-blindness functioned, articulating relations of power to accredit and segment bodies.

The invention of various psychometric tests furthered the problematisation of individuals accredited as abnormal. Difference could now be calculated and inscribed upon the newly formed psychology of the individual. A whole lexicon had been formed through which individuals could be described as normal or abnormal. The emergence of individual psychology across this axis is detailed by Rose (1984: 290–334). The aforementioned tests allowed for the categorising, sorting and segmenting of individuals to be done by increasingly precise means. As detailed in Chapter 4, Broadbent (1872) had assigned different functions and distinct intellectual attributes to particular regions of the brain. Aside from psychology, the area in which the norm was most often utilised was education. In education the norm came to mean the non-problematic. Along this shared axis of the norm a relation was instituted between psychology and education. Nikolas Rose shows how the modern psychology of the individual was formed in the early twentieth century around the problem of classifying and educating those accredited as feeble-minded, and how this relationship was crucial to the institutionalisation of psychology (Rose, 1984: particularly 251–334). The education of those children accredited as backward and defective was typically viewed as a hopeless task. With results being difficult to achieve, the task was considered by Hinshelwood to be arduous (1907: 1232 makes it clear that this is how the undiagnosed congenitally word-blind are perceived). The writers discussed in the following were thus involved in a double process of differentiation: the subjects needed to be established as abnormal so that alternative or intensive teaching methods could be deployed upon them. Yet, equally, those same subjects had to be established as not being backward or defective so that their education was not considered to be a hopeless and ultimately pointless task.

Nettleship (1901) noted that after reading Hinshelwood (1900a) he revisited several cases he had previously encountered, realising that this newly established diagnostic category described the attributes he had found in these children. Nettleship describes the utility of the diagnosis as a way of distinguishing between different groups within the broader category of backward and defective children:

The education of 'backward' and 'defective' children, by more or less special methods, is already receiving more attention than formerly. If from amongst such children, those can be sifted whose only, or principal difficulty is real inability to learn to read, the result cannot be useful both to the individuals and the community. (1901: 67)

Here, a distinction is being drawn between backward and defective children and those whose principle difficulty is in reading. Nevertheless, unlike many of the other papers discussed in what follows (Hinshelwood, 1902, 1904; Thomas, 1905), children accredited with congenital word-blindness are still seen to fall broadly under the category of the backward and defective. Intelligence was being positioned here as a multi-faceted phenomenon constituted by various attributes. The process of sifting through backward and defective children to find those whose only principle difficulty was with reading texts allowed for a section of the population, typically considered to be hopeless in regard to their educatability, to be seen in a new light as people worthy of, and receptive to, education. Congenital word-blindness functioned as a technology of great utility because it was able to sift through those accredited as backward and defective, discerning who could become literate and educated subjects. Similar diagnoses had also been made possible, as particular attributes of intelligence had been assigned to different regions of the brain (Broadbent, 1872). Nettleship situates this technology among a growing interest in the appropriate strategies for educating those accredited as either backward or defective. The usefulness of this technology of power was made apparent by a growing interest in acting upon the bodies of those accredited as backward and defective (Nettleship, 1901: 67).

Hinshelwood, as shall be described in the section 'Defending the Borders', was concerned with protecting the boundaries of the diagnosis and the specificity of its use (Gieryan, 1983). By maintaining the specificity of the diagnosis, he helped to sustain his particular image of the diagnosis and thus keep it under his auspice. An unambiguous and definite diagnosis was a potentially more useful technology of differentiation than a wide category that could encompass vast numbers of people, as it allowed for a distinction to be made through accreditation and to be enunciated onto a precise population at a loud volume. Maintaining a precise operation for congenital word-blindness was therefore an attempt to maintain its utility as a technology of power. The technology served to vociferously proclaim the difference between those diagnosed as congenitally word-blind from two groups: those who are accredited as normal and those accredited as backward. For

Hinshelwood it was important that *not* every child who exhibited a difficulty with reading, even for reasons seemingly cerebral in their origin, was diagnosed as congenitally word-blind. The difficulty had to be of a sufficient degree:

> With regard to diagnosis, I would point out in the first place that every case of inability to learn to read is not necessarily a case of 'congenital word-blindness.' A short time ago, a child was brought to me who after being two years at school did not know the letters of the alphabet, and it was therefore suspected there must be something wrong with its eyesight. On examination I found this inability to learn the letters was not due to any defect of vision but to a cerebral cause, and yet I did not regard it was as belonging to that category which I have described as 'congenital word-blindness.' On careful examination I found that all the forms of memory were defective. The child was not only unable to learn anything by heart. His mother could not trust him to perform the simplest message correctly. Not only were all the forms of memory defective. The inability to learn to read was not in this case due to any local, but to a general failure of cerebral development; hence it did not come under the category of cases described by the term 'congenital word-blindness.' (1902: 94–5)

Word-blindness, as discussed in Chapter 4, could only be diagnosed if there was no evidence of problems with vision, so there was no doubt in the cerebral origin of the difficulty (see the discussion in Chapter 3). The origins of the difficulty had to be cerebral. The differentiation of those diagnosed as congenitally word-blind from the backward and defective was Hinshelwood's concern. The case in question could be identified as backward or defective, as the origin of this accredited difficulty was understood to be cerebral. Congenital word-blindness had to be a local cerebral failure as distinguished from a more general cerebral failure. This organisation of a subject's intellectual abilities into local areas, which could, in turn, be distinguished from a general failure, relies upon Hinshelwood's earlier work on mind-blindness (1900b) and Broadbent's (1872) proposal that certain regions of the brain were responsible for specific functions. A child diagnosed with congenital word-blindness could therefore have only one form of defective memory, while children understood as backward and defective were seen to have difficulty in all these areas. The subject is also not awarded the diagnosis of congenital word-blindness if he is unable to learn anything by heart. While this is shown by Hinshelwood as evidence of a general, rather than local, defect, it also evidences the emphasis on curability that Hinshelwood would soon add to the diagnostic criteria (see the following and Hinshelwood, 1902: 94–5). This case functioned to alert physicians that congenital word-blindness was to be reserved for a very specific group: those who are intelligent in other respects apart from their difficulty with reading, but whose reading difficulty is of a sufficiently severe degree. The notion of degrees of severity became a crucial component in the operation of congenital word-blindness as a technology of power.

The schoolmaster testimonial presented by Hinshelwood (1904: 400–1) isolated the boy's educational difficulties as being only with reading, stating that in other subjects he was at least average and often above the expected standard (Hinshelwood, 1904: 400–1). The isolation of particular attributes was paramount to the possibility of this diagnosis. The isolation of the boy's educational difficulties as only being a problem with a single attribute—reading—enacted a process of differentiation where the boy was distinguished from the population who were accredited as backward and defective children. The segmentation of intelligence into various attributes made it possible for individuals to excel in some areas, but to be considered backward in others (Broadbent, 1872). Diagnoses such as amusia and congenital word-blindness were responses to this sectioned view of the human brain. The uniqueness, rareness and peculiarity of the case is made apparent as the teacher is said to not have seen anything like this in twenty-five years of teaching (Hinshelwood, 1904: 400–1). This raises the question of why such cases, or at least similar cases, would become so prevalent in the coming years, and creates a conceptual tension with Hinshelwood (1896, 1900a, 1904) and Nettleship (1901), who both rallied against the rarity of the diagnosis.

> I wrote to his schoolmaster for information about the boy. He replied that the lad had experienced through his whole career in the school the greatest difficulty in learning to read, which had kept him very much behind in his progress through the school. He was strong in arithmetic, good at spelling, and average in other subjects, including geography and history. 'I have never' said his teacher, 'seen a case similar to this one in my 25 years experience as a teacher. There is another boy in his class, who is quite a poor reader, but this boy is all-around poor, showing no sign of smartness in anything.' (Hinshelwood, 1904: 400–1)

The emphasis upon the uniqueness and rarity of the symptoms acts to differentiate the boy from a larger mass of children who could be encompassed under the category of 'backward' or 'defective'. The process of differentiation is continued as it is established that this boy should not be understood in the same bracket as another in the same class who, while being a poor reader, showed no 'smartness in anything' (Hinshelwood, 1904: 400–1). The boy's educational difficulties had to be localised to the skill of reading—they could not be general. The necessity of distinguishing those understood as being congenitally 'word-blind' from the 'feeble-minded' is thus apparent. Showing evidence of intelligence in a particular area was the virtue that distinguished children accredited with congenital word-blindness from the population accredited as backward or defective.

Thomas establishes that the cerebral make-up of children accredited with congenital word-blindness is different to those considered to be normal (1905: 380). This is achieved through the deployment of research that had been conducted in neurology and specifically around memory (such as the research conducted by his mentor Hinshelwood on mind-blindness (1900b), and Broadbent (1872)). Thomas asserts that 'most adults are found to fall into one or other of the definite memory types—audial, visual or motor' (1905: 380). This shows that cerebral make-up is now being conceived of as varying, even though it is invisible to the human eye; humans are being understood as having dominant and definite memory types. Mapping particular intellectual and educational abilities onto particular regions of the brain was initially conducted by Broadbent (1872) and reiterated by Hinshelwood (1900b). This constituted a new layer of human difference made visible through the deployment of neurological technologies to describe the functioning of memory. From this point on, as a result of this newly constituted diagram, the population could be segmented along the lines of their definite memory type. The sectoring of the brain facilitates the segmentation of the population; it is able to generalise the operation of power from the individual to the population (Ewald, 1990, 1991). Thomas's (1905) work illustrates how new psychological, neurological or medical knowledge established a new image of the individual and, in turn, of the population. In Thomas's (1905) papers this new image was deployed to reconfigure an existing diagnosis in light of these developments, further facilitating the reorganisation of the population. Congenital word-blindness became, in diagnostic terms, simply an exaggeration of the dominance of one type of memory that Thomas believed to be in all individuals (Thomas, 1905: 380). The fashioning of diagnostic categories, such as congenital word-blindness, alters the diagram of the 'normal human', albeit it in small, but precise, ways as further layers from which an individual can deviate from the norm are produced.

The discussion in this and the second half of Chapter 4 evidences that congenital word-blindness was engineered as a technology that could differentiate between those children who, apart from their inability to read, seemed bright or were, indeed, highly intelligent from those who seemingly had difficulties in most of their educational pursuits. It was a diagnosis that served to establish a difference between a specific localised educational difficulty and a general educational difficulty. The need to allow children who had a severe difficulty with reading, but were otherwise quite bright, to become useful bodies seems to have been the driving force behind the development of the diagnostic category of congenital word-blindness. It was necessary that these individuals were differentiated from other children for two reasons. First, so that the study of children accredited congenital word-blindness could define that category's conceptual limits, so that it would be an area of discussion separate to that of the study of 'backward' children. Second, so that the possibility of 'curing' those children accredited with congenital word-blindness of their condition could be established, or at least so that the medical profession could provide advice on how these children should be educated.

The establishment of the possibility to educate some children differently to the majority, but with the same goal of achieving a distinct kind of subjectivity, suggests that the educational system desired to produce a certain type of body.[1] Strategies for education needed to sort between those whose work would be based upon the use of their bodies, and those whose work would be based upon the use of their minds. Children accredited with congenital word-blindness were perceived as having an exaggerated dominance of a particular memory type and after specific interventions were able to attain abilities and skills that were economically desirable. Those who would usually be expected, owing to their affluent background or high intellect, to be involved in work that would use their minds but, owing to their inability to read, were hampered from doing so, could now be educated by altered and specialised methods. Skills could be fostered in bodies previously understood to be beyond the reach of the machineries of government. A rationality for rectifying some defective bodies through segregated or specialised education had been formed, and an assemblage of a variety of technologies of government was being formulated to achieve its goals.

Attempts to prove that a diagnosed child could be highly advanced, perhaps even the most intelligent child in the peer group, but could lack the ability to read, made up a large proportion of the cases presented by Hinshelwood. The child accredited with congenital word-blindness had to be defined as different from educationally backward children so that he or she could receive additional help or allowances, but also so that men like Hinshelwood could justify their research. There was little interest in giving children who had difficulty without a specific pathology, or those who were seen as having no hope of improving their educational attainment, any extra educational provisions.

One is Deserving if One Can be Cured

In every case which I have met with up to the present, the children have been taught to read, and my experience has been borne out by that of others. (Hinshelwood, 1907: 1231)

Differentiating bodies from both those accredited as normal and those accredited as backward and defective, has been established above as a key operation performed by congenital word-blindness. A theme present throughout all the papers discussed within this chapter (excluding Rutherford, 1909) is the deserving nature of the subjects diagnosed with congenital word-blindness. By deserving I mean that the subjects are presented in a sympathetic fashion—with teachers, parents and the examiners extolling their intelligence, their good character and even good looks (Hinshelwood, 1902: 93–4, 1907: 1230; Minogue, 1927: 226). Accounts are given of how many of the patients have achieved careers which would be considered to be successful, for example an account is given of a patient who became a lawyer (Nettleship, 1901: 64). This possibility of the subjects being cured or overcoming congenital word-blindness appears to mark them as deserving. Children accredited with congenital word-blindness deserve to be differentiated from backward and defective children because, as the cases illustrate, after years of precisely directed educational intervention they could become some of the most successful members of society (Hinshelwood, 1896, 1900a, 1902, 1907; Thomas, 1905; Nettleship, 1901). We shall now continue the discussion of the process of differentiation discussed above, but move away from the technical aspect of this process towards a discussion of the moral values that were attached to bodies by this operation. The value attached to the bodies is that of 'deserving'. My analysis here draws upon Davis's (1995) concept of a deserving defect, the notion that some differences accredited as defects were imbued with moral characteristics which framed them as deserving. Those diagnosed with congenital word-blindness were considered to be deserving, therefore distinguishing them from the population accredited as backward and defective, and who were marked as undeserving.

An example of how the diagnosis was framed as deserving can be seen in Nettleship (1901), where he offers an example of how the patients he subsequently diagnosed attained successful careers after their education had been diverted onto a different path. Here, he informs us that one of the patients he saw has now become a lawyer (Nettleship, 1901: 64). Respectable, highly-paid careers that require the individual to have achieved a high level of education are thus still within the grasp of the children diagnosed as congenitally word-blind. The adjusted teaching methods discussed have thus been successful in creating productive *bodies* from these *bodies* that were hitherto considered to be backward and defective.

In his 1902 paper Hinshelwood provides details of two case studies of patients he had recently encountered. These discussions provide further evidence of how the diagnosed were being framed as deserving. The descriptions of the patients once again assert how the subjects in question should be understood as curable and deserving. The first case details the gravity of difficulty in reading, but it also illustrates the subject's strong desire to be educated:

> So great was her difficulty in learning it that at times it seemed an impossibility, and on several occasions her mother abandoned the task in despair. She was however returned to it again and again, and after nine months labour she learned although imperfectly, the letters of the alphabet, though even yet she makes occasional mistakes in naming the letters. (1902: 92)

The description of the second case focuses on intelligence and how a boy was able to utilise his intelligence in other areas to conceal the defect for a while:

> He was pushed on for a time with the other children, because he successfully concealed the fact of his inability to read, by learning his reading lesson by heart. His mother says that he is a smart intelligent boy, even smarter and quicker in many respects then her other children, his one defect according to her being that he cannot be taught to read. (1902: 93–4)

The first case describes the persistence of both the patient and the educator towards the girl's education, which resulted in an immense improvement in the girl's reading. This may not show the curability of those accredited as congenitally word-blind, but it does show how their skills with reading can be, with carefully directed instruction, improved. In the second case the notable intelligence of the boy who will be accredited as congenitally word-blind is established, presenting him as perhaps even more intelligent, at least in some respects, than his siblings. Curability and perceived intelligence are qualities that distinguish these two cases from the subject (discussed above and found in Hinselwood, 1902: 94–5) who Hinshelwood felt was not suitable for the congenital word-blindness diagnosis. Congenital word-blindness is thus a diagnosis for generally intelligent subjects who have a localised specific difficulty with a single attribute of intelligence. It is this contrast between general intelligence and a local difficulty that marks those designated as congenitally word-blind as deserving. As the teaching methods discussed in the next section will show, this general intelligence was to be used as the basis for training methods that would alleviate the problems engendered by word-blindness.

Advocating an Early Diagnosis

Amongst the many criteria proposed for successfully training children who have been accredited as congenitally word-blind, the advocacy of an early diagnosis was, perhaps, the most commonly favoured strategy of correction. This championing of early diagnosis comes as no surprise, as it is evident that Hinshelwood conceives of the lack of a widely known and established diagnosis to be a moral predicament that requires a hasty reconciliation:

> It is evident that it is a matter of the highest importance to recognise as early as possible the true nature of this defect, when it is met with in a child. It may prevent much waste of valuable time and may save the child from suffering and cruel treatment. (1902: 97–8)

The diagnosis is viewed by Hinshelwood as an apparatus to stop intelligent children being misinterpreted as feeble-minded, and as a means to protect them against unjust and cruel treatment. The statement concerning children being misinterpreted as 'stupid' or 'lazy' is restated by Hinshelwood (1902: 97–8), who also critiques the lack of training methods for children accredited as congenitally word-blind. Hinshelwood

(1902) suggests that because techniques for training children accredited with congenital word-blindness are not proliferated widely throughout the educational system, these children are often subjected to unfair treatment. This value judgement of relative fairness positions those children diagnosed with congenital word-blindness as deserving. Like Nettleship (1901), Hinshelwood (1902) is concerned about the loss of the most malleable period of children's lives and wishes to avoid potentially important educational resources being misdirected. He wants to make sure that the most favourable teaching techniques for the particular pupils are deployed at the optimal period. The deserving character of these children situates the educational system's lack of techniques for instructing them as a moral failing. Hinshelwood's diagnosis is therefore working in assemblage with the philanthropic calls to educate the population as a method of institutionalising the diagnosis.

An example of this moral failing is illustrated with a description of how children accredited with a reading difficulty had hitherto been perceived as either stupid or lazy: 'When a child manifests great difficulty in learning to read and is unable to keep up in progress with its fellows, the cause is generally assigned to stupidity or laziness, and no systematized method is directed to the training of such a child' (1902: 98). The norm here is being articulated into the activity of education. If an individual is unable to keep up to standards derived from measuring the attributes against their peers, then they are problematised. It is this child's inability to seemingly keep up with his peers that is being problematised: 'the child would then be regarded in the proper light as one with a congenital defect in a particular area of the brain, a defect which, however, can often be remedied by persevering and persistent training' (1902: 98). Children previously considered as lazy or backward could now, through the deployment of specialised methods of instruction, be taught and their educational difficulties overcome. The mapping of precise intellectual attributes onto specific regions of the brain made it possible to articulate a localised defect or, in the more positive terms of Thomas (1905), a dominant memory type, as the aetiology for a diagnosis. Technologies of power were able to refine from a multitude of bodies considered to be uneducatable, an array of bodies that could, in fact, receive instruction. One of the operations congenital word-blindness performed was to act as a filter.

Descriptions of the brain have been a feature of the writings on reading difficulties since Broadbent (1872). Hinshelwood continually used this material as a point of departure to take his version of the diagnosis

in a new direction. A call for an early diagnosis is advocated, again utilising description of the brain, to suggest that the chances for 'overcoming' the difficulty are better earlier in a child's life:

> The sooner the true nature of the defect is recognised, the better
> are the chances of the child's improvement. In the early period of
> life the brain cells and fibres are more capable of marked develop-
> ment than in the later periods, and hence the earlier the systematic
> training of the individual the better the chances of overcoming the
> difficulty. (1902: 98)

Hinshelwood considers the brain to respond better to attempts to cultivate it in earlier life rather than in later life. The earlier a diagnosis is
made in the patient's life the greater the chance of them responding to
intervention. A specific method for teaching children accredited with
congenital word-blindness to read is then proposed. This practice takes
advantage of the localised character of congenital word-blindness:

> I have recommended in such cases the use of sets of block letters.
> This enables the child to assist the visual memory by the sense of
> touch. When it has mastered the letters, it can then arrange these
> into words. The sense of touch seems to give some real assistance to
> the weakened visual memory in retaining the visual impressions.
> (1902: 98)

The technique described above relies on Hinshelwood's earlier work
(1900b), which had, in turn, built upon Broadbent (1872), and which
separated memory into different components: visual memory, audial
memory and kinaesthetic memory. Kinaesthetic memory is used to
assist in developing a skill typically associated with visual memory.
It is assumed that by deploying techniques that utilise other types of
memory, fertile conditions for educating the subjects in question can be
fostered. This is reliant upon considering congenital word-blindness to
be a localised difficulty, connected to an accredited deficiency in one
region of the brain. The solution is simply to deploy different regions of
the brain to compensate for this difficulty. The conditions necessary for
training are then described:

> There is no use of attempting to teach such children reading in a
> class along with other children with normally developed brains. The
> contrast between their difficulty and the facility of the other will

only discourage them. Such children must be taught separately by special methods adapted to help them overcome their difficulties. (Hinshelwood, 1902: 98–9)

Segregating children accredited with congenital word-blindness is thus presented as being in their interests as it will protect them from unfair treatment and discouragement. The segregative educational rationale was promoted owing to the perceived under-development of the subject's brain. The proposed segmenting of the population had now moved beyond articulating a medical diagnosis to ascribe a sign onto the body; the diagnosis was now being articulated into the machinery of segmenting educational populations. Attributing particular functions onto different regions of the brain facilitated the segmentation of different children along the lines of localised defects. Children with normally developed brains were positioned as the site upon which mainstream education aimed to act; the brain had become the site from which educational normality is derived. This assemblage of technologies concerned with describing the brain and the norm allowed for individual characteristics to be articulated as attributes of a certain 'kind' of person—qualities that would be found in a normal individual. The technology of norm here allowed for the generalising of power from the individual body to the body of a population (Ewald, 1990, 1991). Hinshelwood alerts teachers that they should not be discouraged or fall to the temptation of viewing the task of teaching such children as hopeless. He claims that 'experience has taught us that persistence and persevering attempts will often overcome difficulties which at first sight seem insuperable' (Hinshelwood, 1902: 99). Sympathy is shown for those teachers who find teaching these pupils frustrating; they are encouraged not to be deterred, as persistence has been a successful factor in previous cases. Attempts are being made to establish categories of children that, despite their accredited difficulties, can still attain acceptable levels of education through the deployment of specialist techniques. One of these categories was congenital word-blindness.

A paramount concern for Hinshelwood was ensuring that teachers did not give up on the possibility of educating these pupils. He tried to persuade teachers that through the deployment of the correct techniques, children accredited as congenitally word-blind can become successful and productive subjects, as long as the modified teaching methods were deployed at an early enough point in the child's life (1902: 99). Once educationalists understood how to deploy it, children whose educational prospects were considered to be hopeless could be understood anew. This acted to transform how a part of the educational populace was understood. It facilitated the flowing of power by establishing capillaries to sites that were previously less porous to the activity of government. In doing so it allowed attributes to be proliferated throughout a set of bodies that had previously been seen as unable to develop skills such as literacy. This diagnosis could be deployed by various rationalities of government, but its formation seems to have occurred under the influence of the rationales of government concerned with perfecting bodies and cultivating the population. Congenital word-blindness seems to embody two aspects of bio-politics: (1) treating bodies as capital; and (2) segmenting the individual body and the body of the population into units. Thus, in one small technology of power the dominant characteristics of bio-politics are encompassed.

Training and Education

Hinshelwood (1902, 1904: 405) and his associate Thomas (1905) called for the compulsory examination of all children accredited as defective, backward or feeble-minded so that they could be properly organised into various groups. Some of these smaller populations had a greater hope of benefiting from specialist educational techniques than others. Compulsory examination of all children accredited as defective would allow the diagnosis to be applied to a larger number of bodies. If all children believed to be defective were examined, the character of their difficulties could be analysed, allowing in some cases for specialist techniques to be deployed which would help them overcome a localised difficulty such as congenital word-blindness. The compulsory examination of all children accredited as defective, the diagnosis of congenital word-blindness and the corresponding specialist teaching methods were all part of a machinery of government that could operate in assemblage with a variety of other technologies to sift through bodies accredited as backward and defective. This machinery of government operated to identify those who could, in fact, be trained through the deployment of specialist teaching methods.

Specialised educational techniques could be deployed once children accredited as congenitally word-blind had been differentiated from those accredited as defective, backward or feeble-minded. The likelihood of these techniques being successful was considered to be greater if an early diagnosis had been made (Bruner, 1905: 195; Hinshelwood, 1902: 97–8; Jackson, 1906: 848 reiterated this sentiment). Compulsory

examination would facilitate early diagnosis and allow the specialist teaching techniques to be deployed earlier, allowing intervention
to begin when the brain is considered to be at its most malleable.
Hinshelwood described methods that could be utilised to transform the
children accredited as defective who were then diagnosed with congenital word-blindness into productive bodies:

> I have, therefore, insisted on the fact that all these children should
> be taught alone and not in a class along with other children with
> normally developed brains. The contrast between their own diffi-
> culty and the comparative ease with which other children learn to
> read is a constant source of discouragement both to themselves and
> to their teachers. The task is abandoned as hopeless, and such chil-
> dren often leave school without being able to read, as in the case
> of the two elder boys recorded in this paper. The case of the oldest
> boy is especially instructive. He left school, after being seven years
> there, without being able to read. He could not then even read the
> simplest child's primer. Since then he has educated himself by four
> years steady persevering effort, and can now read a little, although
> very imperfectly as yet. (1907: 1232)

The appropriate method for teaching children accredited as being congenitally word-blind is thus argued to be isolation. This protects both
the children and the teachers, ensuring that they will not abandon the
pursuit of learning themselves or be disregarded as a hopeless case. The
process of segmentation taking place is complex, as those classified as
congenitally word-blind are to be distinguished from two groups: those
accredited with having normal brains and those identified as being
feeble-minded, backward or defective. Unlike those accredited as
defective, the congenitally word-blind are understood as being able to
improve, moving within (or at least very close to) the boundaries demar-
cated by the norm. Hinshelwood's account of the boy, who through his
own seemingly unrelenting dedication to the task has educated himself, positions this boy, and those accredited as congenitally word-blind
more generally, as having a deserving defect (Davis, 1995). The deserving character of those accredited with congenital word-blindness positions these bodies as requiring the attention of specific technologies
of power. Attitudes concerning training and education were formed a
few years after the diagnosis had been invented; a slight shift in these
occurs with Thomas's (1905) insertion of the hereditary hypothesis into
the clinical machinery.

The Insertion of the Hereditary Hypothesis

According to Hinshelwood (1907), the most important innovation regarding reading difficulties since his own pioneering research is the insertion of the hereditary hypothesis into the diagnosis by Thomas (1905). This recalibration of the technology engenders a distinct shift in the bio-political positions of Hinshelwood and a new consensus on several issues being established. In this section the insertion of the hereditary hypothesis into the diagnostic machinery is described. Furthermore, I will also consider how this affected the functioning of the diagnosis at a minute, technical level and in its potential interactions with the wider activities of government.

Thomas draws upon evidence of congenital word-blindness occurring among several members of the same family in numerous cases to assert that the diagnosis may assume a family type. He notes, moreover, that this tendency is likely to be found in the allied conditions of *idioglossia, amusia* and congenital deafness. This similarity in memory types is akin to the research findings of Broadbent (1872) and Hinshelwood (1895). Relations between these various conditions are here further sedimented. Congenital word-blindness is starting to be situated in a cosmology of educational conditions that are understood to take a family type and to be specific, rather than general, defects. The wide category of backward and defective children is being split and segmented into several more precise groupings, where education is no longer necessarily seen as hopeless (Thomas, 1905: 381). For a child accredited as defective to be separated from those for whom there is no hope of educating, their defect must be discovered to be local to one region of the brain as techniques for educating localised defects had been established.

The connection between different family members implies not only that congenital word-blindness is given an organic origin, but that it is seen as familial and hereditary. Supplying the diagnosis an organic origin increased the diagnosis's veritable character, as it became a physical difference that could be seen through the application of the correct lens to medicine's microscopic toolkit. A familial aetiology established the characteristics that congenital word-blindness was concerned with, and was seen by some as existing within the individual's family history, even before the body in question was born. There seem to be two distinct ways of interpreting this. First, the pre-existence of these characteristics in a family's past further establishes the deserving nature of children accredited with congenital word-blindness, as the defect is engendered by a factor prior to them, or, second, a relation could be made here to the eugenicist's concern with the degeneration of the stock of the population (Hasian, 1996: 35).

Hinshelwood's 'Four Cases of Word-blindness in the Same Family' (1907) utilised Thomas' (1905) paper to elaborate and expand his conception of word-blindness. Thomas's paper is viewed by Hinshelwood to be of considerable importance, perhaps the most important development in the area of the study since his own work, as it proposes that that congenital word-blindness is likely to occur among family groups (Thomas, 1905: 381). Hinshelwood was keen to acknowledge his own success, and the innovative and prestigious nature of his previous research (Hinshelwood, 1907: 1230), detailing how congenital word-blindness was now a recognised diagnostic category in both Britain and the USA. For instance, Hinshelwood states that 'knowledge of this subject has gradually been diffused amongst ophthalmologists':

> Since this communication there have been numerous cases reported in this country, in America, and on the Continent, but with one exception nothing has been added to the further elucidation of the subject, beyond what I stated in my Lancet article on May 26th, 1900. The exception to which I refer is the paper by Dr. C. J. Thomas, Assistant Medical Officer, London County Council, which appeared in the Ophthalmic Review, August, 1905. In this paper Dr. Thomas called special attention to the fact that congenital word-blindness may assume a family type and that a hereditary tendency is probable. The present example of four members of the same family with congenital word-blindness is a brilliant confirmation of the correctness of Dr. Thomas's observation. (1907: 1230)

This keenness to acknowledge the diffusion of the diagnosis amongst ophthalmologists and its recognition as a legitimate diagnosis in both the UK and the USA gives further weight to the argument that Hinshelwood was concerned with the institutionalisation of the diagnosis. Hinshelwood explains how the four boys in this family were brought to see him. His account illustrates how coming into contact with a physician versed in the specifics of congenital word-blindness was the most likely way for a prospective patient to be diagnosed. This was owing to the fact that the compulsory examination of children accredited as defective was not yet in place. The diagnosis was only articulated onto bodies that were taken to a clinic[2] where compulsory examination would institute a wide variety of capillaries allowing the diagnosis to be inscribed onto bodies that would not have come to the clinic of any expert in congenital word-blindness, such as Hinshelwood or Thomas. The account informs us that it was by personal arrangement that the four boys in this family were brought to Hinshelwood:

> Mr. Heard informed me that there was no difficulty experienced in the education of the first seven members of the family, but that the eighth, ninth, tenth, and eleventh—all boys—experienced the greatest difficulties in learning to read. He also said that in his long experience as a teacher he had never before met with anything like the difficulties encountered in attempting to teach these four boys to read, and that he was greatly puzzled by how to account for it, as in every other respect the boys seemed so intelligent. Dr. W. Lewis Thomson, Assistant Medical Officer of Health for Lanarkshire, to whom he had mentioned the remarkable case of the four boys, at once recognized the true nature of the difficulty. Dr. Thomson, being an old pupil of my own, was thoroughly conversant with the nature of congenital word-blindness, and at once recognizing that the four boys were typical cases of this condition, kindly arranged that the children should be sent to see me. (1907: 1230)

Professional networks appear to be important in the diagnosis of children as congenitally word-blind because knowledge of the diagnosis has been dispersed through them (note Thomas's relationship with Hinshelwood, or Stephenson's position as the editor of *Ophthalmoscope*, for example). Without the compulsory examination of children accredited as defective the diagnosis could only be inscribed onto a very limited population—those who came directly in contact with experts. Positions of influence allowed the diagnosis to disperse into a wider array of capillaries. For example, Stephenson's editorship of the *Ophthalmoscope* provided a platform for much research on the topic to be published and support at conferences to be voiced. Thomas's position as Assistant Medical Officer for Lanarkshire also made the case for compulsory examination louder. These positions of influence were of great importance to the diagnosis gaining institutional acceptance.

Again, we are informed via a teacher's testimony that these children were in all ways, apart from their difficulty with reading, 'normal'. Again, this emphasises how the isolation of this single 'ability' as defective was a key characteristic of congenital word-blindness. It had to be a localised difficulty, as the foretasted arguments by Hinshelwood had claimed. Apart from establishing the occurrence of congenital word-blindness in one family, and thus furthering the hypothesis that it may be hereditary, there is little else of unique or noteworthy character in Hinshelwood's descriptions of the cases in this article. The occurrence within a single family implies a biological familial relation that adds further credence to the organic aetiology that Thomas (1905) and Hinshelwood (1900a, 1902, 1904) had been concerned with establishing:

> The four cases of congenital word-blindness recorded in this paper present no new aspects if taken individually, but the record of four consecutive cases occurring in the same family is unique, so far as I am aware. It affords the strongest confirmation of the important observation made by Dr. C. J. Thomas in the papers previously quoted, that congenital word-blindness frequently assumes a family type, and that a hereditary tendency is probable. The four boys affected were the youngest members of a family of eleven, and the seven older members all learned to read without experiencing any abnormal difficulty. The striking point about the cases of the four boys is their close resemblance to each other, showing that the cerebral defect in each case was very similar. In other respects than the great difficulty experienced in learning to read, these four boys were quite as intelligent as the other members of the family. They all learned to count fairly well. Their memory, except for the visual memory of words and letters, was good. They all learned to write easily, and could copy correctly and well. It is evident that their cerebral defect was a purely local one, and also very similar in each case, in short, that it was strictly confined to the cerebral area for the visual memory of words and letters, the left angular gyrus, and did not extend at all beyond that. (Hinshelwood, 1907: 1231)

The hereditary origin is stressed by describing the physical resemblances between the four boys: their physical likeness is presented as further evidence of the familial connection. They are presented as being as intelligent as other members of the family apart from their difficulty with reading. The localised quality of congenital word-blindness, which further specifies that the characteristics are contained in the left angular gyrus, is maintained after the insertion of the hereditary hypothesis into the diagnostic machinery. Hinshelwood adopts a cautionary tone, alerting his fellow ophthalmologists to the care they must take when diagnosing individuals as congenitally word-blind. Hinshelwood iterates the localised character of the difficulty, and their deservingness as key components of the diagnostic machinery, by stating that the patient must in all other ways be as intelligent as other children. Distinguishing between those accredited as backward, defective or feeble-minded, and those who, as we know from Hinshelwood's previous writings, are to be considered as deserving of special treatment and education, was of paramount concern (1896: 1508). Misdiagnosis must be avoided. This process of differentiation—which sorts, segments and marks bodies—is made possible by a variety of technologies, including the norm operating in the assemblage. Congenital word-blindness forms part of a particular machinery of government for segmenting and differentiating between the educational multitude, establishing distinct populations who can be acted upon differently. At a technical level it must also be noted that Hinshelwood seems to be protecting the boundaries of the diagnosis that he has paid a crucial role in establishing, so that it will not be utilised to misinterpret the character of children accredited as feeble-minded:

> In the diagnosis of such cases also attention must be paid to the general intelligence of the patient. Congenital word-blindness is a local affection of the brain, and such patients, as a rule, are as bright and intelligent as other children. In the 4 cases under consideration the boys in other respects were quite as intelligent as the other seven members of the family. Such cases must be carefully distinguished from those where there is, in addition to difficulty in learning to read, a general lack of intelligence and general failure of the mental powers. In this latter group the difficulty in learning to read is due to a general lack of development of the higher cerebral centres, and should not be mistaken for congenital word-blindness, which is an affection of a special cerebral area in an otherwise normal and healthy brain. (1907: 1231)

The process of establishing differences between those children accredited as word-blind from those accredited as being feeble-minded is strengthened here as Hinshelwood deploys neurological knowledge to produce a difference between the brains of congenitally word-blind children and children accredited as being feeble-minded. This function of differentiation is achieved by again stressing the localised failure of a part of the brain in congenitally word-blind children on the one hand, and the general failure of the entire brain in backward and defective children on the other.[3] This increases the organic character of both the differences in question, and, in addition, furthers the conceptual, technical and organisational distance between them. This process of separating children accredited as congenitally word-blind from those accredited as feeble-minded also crucially marks congenitally word-blind children as deserving and the feeble-minded as undeserving. The process of segmenting the population is facilitated by the mapping of particular intellectual abilities onto specific regions of the brain. This process of segmentation had an associated function of establishing moral values of deservingness and un-deservingness onto the bodies of those bodies, which came to be described by particular diagnostic categories.

An American Challenge

Within the borders of the UK, Hinshelwood's vision of the diagnosis appears to have claimed institutional acceptance, with articles by him or those who followed his vision being published in prestigious journals (both specialist journals, e.g. *Ophthalmoscope* (Hinshelwood, 1904) and *Ophthalmic Review* (Hinshelwood, 1902), and those directed at a more general medical audience, e.g. *The Lancet* (Hinshelwood, 1900a) and the *British Medical Journal* (Hinshelwood, 1907)). Hinshelwood's work is also cited continually as *the* point of reference for the topic (Bruner (1905), Fisher (1905), Nettleship (1901) and Thomas (1905) all use Hinshelwood work as their key point of departure), a position that important figures (Stephen Stephenson, editor of *Ophthalmoscope*) give their patronage and support to. Hinshelwood's conception of the diagnosis was not so well received in continental Europe (Wernickle in Claiborne, 1906; Wernickle in Hinshelwood, 1904) or in the USA (Jackson, 1906; Rutherford, 1909). Criticisms were presented regarding his use of terminology and some of his clinical hypotheses. The sets of terms and concepts linked to different players relate to different conceptions of the diagnosis and different political agendas. This becomes relatively obvious in the following discussion of Rutherford's distinct terminology and political persuasion, and represents a grappling for jurisdiction over the diagnosis and a way to distinguish his work from the dominant mode of considering it, which, at this juncture, was Hinshelwood's. Challenging terminology rather than clinical data may have been the easiest way to draw attention to a piece of research, showing how the newest research is distinct, innovative and important without having to depart that much from the basics of the diagnosis.

The programme of developing technologies, tactics and strategies for the treatment of those who had been accredited with congenital word-blindness crossed the Atlantic and was taken up by the first American to write on the subject, Edward Jackson (1906). Jackson took issue with the term congenital word-blindness. asserting that it was unscientific.[4] Like several researchers before him, he problematised the visual elements implied in the terminology (Broadbent, 1872, 1896; Wernickle in Claiborne, 1906; Wernickle in Hinshelwood, 1904); 'Congenital word blindness is the term used by Hinshelwood and others to indicate inability or great difficulty in learning to read. The term seems inappropriate for a condition that exists with normal visual acuteness and normal fields of vision' (1906: 843). He offered an alternative and, in his view, more scientific term: *developmental alexia*. His paper was the first to be published in an American journal, and reviewed the majority of known cases of congenital word-blindness as a way of introducing the diagnosis to the American medical public. Jackson states that 'In only two of the cases had the patient reached adult life with a very marked degree of alexia remaining' (1906: 849), suggesting that the methods of treatment employed had been an effective strategy in the government of educational difference, and had ultimately engendered the production of the desired type of bodies.

Jackson (1906) is thus proposing a terminologically refined diagnosis, a technology with a recalibrated function that challenges the veritable character of Hinshelwood's formulation and the precession of its operation. The refinement of the terminology associated with a diagnosis should be understood as the recalibration of a technology. Jackson then furthers the precision of his altered diagnostic apparatus by taking issue with Hinshelwood's conception of word-blindness resulting from a delayed development in one part of the brain:

> The condition is essentially a failure of development, or a delayed development of a group of co-ordinations, or a co-ordinating centre essential to the recognition of written or printed characters. The term developmental alexia is, therefore, suggested as most specifically indicating the condition under consideration. (1906: 843)

Jackson again provides an aetiology for developmental alexia that is distinct from that associated with congenital word-blindness. This aetiology also relies upon technologies concerned with the brain. However, Jackson departs from describing the reading difficulty as resulting from a failure of memory with a specific region. Establishing that the reading difficulty in question was a defect localised in only one region of the brain and thus only affected one educational attribute, had been of paramount importance to many of the British writers, particularly Hinshelwood (1902: 94–5, 1907: 1230). Jackson's aetiology relies upon a group of co-ordinations, which still localise the difficulty, but to a group of interacting regions rather than a singular one. Developmental alexia may perform the same operation as congenital word-blindness, but with a crucially different component: a distinct aetiology, allowing it to articulate relations of power in a slightly different manner.

The journal in which Rutherford (1909) chose to publish his article is intriguing. Congenital word-blindness is here affirmed as a diagnosis that has in all cases been attached to children, while acquired word-blindness has, of course, been more associated with adults (Hinshelwood, 1895, 1896; Kussmaul, 1887). The journal's title, *The Journal of Children's Diseases*, also frames word-blindness as a disease, a term that hitherto had not been connected to the diagnosis.

Rutherford (1909) uses Morgan (1896) and Hinshelwood (1900) as his points of departure, as had become typical in the literature.[5] Following Hinshelwood (1907), Rutherford positions Thomas (1905) as being crucially important: 'C. J. Thomas called attention to the fact that this congenital form of word-blindness may assume a family type' (1905: 484). This familial typing would appear to open the diagnosis up to insights of a eugenic character. It would appear that Rutherford became interested in congenital word-blindness precisely because of its familial character. He was particularly concerned with typically eugenic themes (Hasian, 1996: 35), such as inbreeding:

> The family history of the present case here detailed goes still further to prove the aetiological influence of germ-plasm defect, and not merely of this alone but of the effect of in-breeding, in giving rise to congenital word-blindness, or, as it may with propriety be termed, dyslexia congenita. (1909: 484)

Rutherford, for reasons not given in the paper, prefers the term dyslexia congenita to congenital word-blindness. He thus proposes a challenge to the relative hegemony that Hinshelwood's terminological device had achieved. Although it had previously been used by Hinshelwood (1896) to describe a 'peculiar case' of acquired word-blindness, this is the first instance of dyslexia being used to describe congenital word-blindness. Rutherford does not use the term developmental alexia (Jackson, 1906) or congenital symbol amblyopia (Claiborne, 1906) proposed by his fellow countrymen. The term dyslexia must be carefully dissected. In medicine, 'dys' typically means bad; 'lex' refers to reading or language; and 'ia' is a Latin suffix meaning disease or disorder—the literal translation of dyslexia would therefore be 'bad reading disor-der'. The use of the first prefix imbues the diagnosis with a particu-larly negative moral connotation and the suffix provides a similar, but less intense, function. Rutherford's diagnostic device refers negatively to the diagram of the norm, while Hinshelwood engaged positively with it.

Rutherford's description of a teacher's testimony about a child, who he later diagnosed with dyslexia congenita, takes a starkly more nega-tive tone than has thus far been encountered in the literature. The edu-cational characteristics associated with those people whose brains are accredited as normal are being articulated as something these subjects are unable to attain:

> Her teacher compared her deficiency in this direction to that of a boy whom she had formerly taught, who had a general lack of intel-ligence, being an incorrigible dunce in every subject and whose brother is a congenital imbecile. It is significant that while talking to me about this girl she used the word stubborn with regard to her at once correcting herself however, and for my benefit replacing the word stupid. (1909: 485)

Those diagnosed with dyslexia congenita are described as being closer to backward and defective children than those considered to be nor-mal. This is a departure from congenital word-blindness, where the subjects are vociferously differentiated from children considered to be backward and defective. Dyslexia congenita here performs a distinct function to congenital word-blindness by imbuing bodies with a dif-ferent set of moral values. Rutherford describes the subject's family his-tory, which, from the details presented, suggests he must consider to be an extremely important element in the understanding of dyslexia congenita. He describes the difficulty of how the lengths undertaken to obtain the family history shows how important this was to his concep-tion of the diagnosis. The examples he highlights alert us to a eugenic influence on his thinking:

> The full details of the family history are of the greatest interest and were not obtained without considerable difficulty and the exercise of much patience. Her parents and grandparents are quite illiterate and she and her sister are the two youngest out of a family of five chil-dren—all illegitimate. Of these five children the first two were born prematurely and both died in fits, one with at five months old, the

other at the age of fourteen weeks. The third child died, when eleven weeks old of what was described as croup, but which in the light of this history, may quite possibility have been either laryngeal spasm or rapidly fatal ocdema glottidis from a laryngeal neurosis, such as older writers used to term 'internal convulsions.' Their mother has been asthmatic for years, and has recently developed hepatic cirrhosis (without, however, any definite indication of its being of syphilitic origin). Some years ago she was operated on for a pedunculated cancer of the thigh; she also has a parenchymatous goitre, of the existence of which she was totally unaware. She is an only child and is herself illegitimate; by the time she was twenty-five she had no less then three illegitimate children of her own and they were all dead. (1909: 486)

This description makes evident that Rutherford considers dysleixa congenita as the outcome of persistent degeneration in a family's organic material. Descriptions like these had not been present in any previous articles concerned with reading difficulties. Rutherford was therefore forming dyslexia congenita to articulate the goals of different strategies of government to congenital word-blindness. Rutherford goes on to explain his reasoning for presenting such detailed family history, again in a tone that departs from the literature described thus far:

A more perfect example could hardly be wished for to illustrate the effect of defective hereditary material in the causation of dyslexia congenita, and to prove that the cerebral lesion, or localised aplasia as it probably is in these cases, may depend on a cause actually antecedent to the first cell division of the fertilised ovum. That the relatives exhibited varying degenerative manifestations and that some of them may have been in their own way quite estimable members of the community is not to be wondered at; a family tottering to its fall not infrequently—to brows an expression by the stock-breeder—'trows' variants from the common stem now to one side and now to the other, and the well known view of Lombroso may be referred to, that genius (in certain case) may be taken as the product of a rotten stock, 'a true degenerative psychosis' as it has been phrased. (1909: 487)

Rutherford utilises Hinshelwood (1900b) and Thomas (1905) as the points of departure for his thinking, following them both in considering this form of word-blindness to be congenital and hereditary.

However, he departs from the paternalistic tone and vocabulary of Hinshelwood regarding children accredited as congenitally word-blind, and intensifies the hereditary hypothesis proposed in Thomas (1905), amplifying it in a fashion that is unmistakably eugenic. He makes analogies to stockbreeders and rotten stock, connecting congenital differences in this family as proof that dyslexia congenita is connected to 'defective hereditary material'. Rutherford also hypothesises that the aetiology of the cerebral difference in question may be 'antecedent to the first cell division of the fertilised ovum'. By returning to this point in search of an aetiology of the cerebral difference that Hinshelwood had suggested engendered congenital word-blindness, the organic aetiology argument is strengthened and those accredited as congenitally word-blind are further differentiated from those accredited as being normal. Rutherford positions the aetiology at a very early point in his life history. This position is, perhaps, the earliest that can be imagined. With this difference being formed close to the point of conception it is constituted as being a profound and significant difference to those accredited as normal. Dyslexia congenita should be understood as being constituted by removing the aetiological component of congenital word-blindness and replacing it with a eugenic aetiology concerned with defective stock.

Relations are thus instituted between dyslexia congenita and various conditions considered by eugenicists to be undesirable or degenerative. Links are seemingly made between dyslexia congenita and other undesirable conditions, including potentially immoral behaviours such as having children outside wedlock. The biological and moral ancestry of a patient is thus seen as determining their condition. The negative moral values being attached to bodies here are in great contrast to the deservingness that Hinshelwood (1900b), Thomas (1905) and Nettleship (1901) presented. Rutherford's descriptions differ from these writers as they are more concerned with performing a process of differentiating between those accredited with dyslexia congenita and those accredited as being normal, rather than Hinshelwood, who was primarily concerned with enacting a process of differentiating between those accredited with congenital word-blindness and those accredited as feeble-minded. This is a crucial difference in how the two diagnostic categories articulated relations of power in distinct ways:

> The condition is thus seen to be of the nature of a reversion to the pre-civilised type as the result of loss or destruction of certain of the later and more highly specialised determinants in the gametic

idioplasm, and as such it falls in line with many other of the phenomena of atavism. (Rutherford, 1909: 487)

Rutherford's negative description of congenital word-blindness as a 'reversion to a pre-civilised' type is very different to the more paternalistic tone of Hinshelwood et al., who emphasised the possibility of children being misinterpreted as feeble-minded and thus subjected to unfair treatment. The aetiology of the dyslexia developing soon after conception operates in assemblage with Rutherford's notion that these patients are a reversion to a pre-civilised type, and articulates these subjects as being far from normal. Children accredited with congenital word-blindness had been presented as deserving (Hinshelwood, 1900b, 1902). Rutherford's work departs from this again, emphasising the hereditary nature of congenital word-blindness, but in a negative fashion, describing it as an atavistic phenomenon. By relating the diagnosis to a variety of phenomena considered to be degenerative, Rutherford is attempting to insert dyslexia congenitally into a eugenic machinery of government.

A description of how Rutherford imagines images to be stored in the memory of a patient accredited with congenital word-blindness makes reference to the images being distorted. People accredited with congenital word-blindness are therefore positioned by Rutherford having as malfunctioning brains:

> The memories of visual concepts of objects are stored as impressionist pictures in the brain. By education the laborious processes of visual sensation, comparison with the previously stored images in the cortex and psychical recognition are made easier, and are carried on almost with the automatic rapidity of reflex action. In cases of congenital word-blindness even after prolonged training all the laborious steps of the process have to be carried out one by one by one with such visible effort that one might almost think the mental machinery were creaking under the strain. The words never come to be vested with significance in virtue of their shape and the general appearance they present to the eye. (1909: 488)

Rutherford's description of the possibility of those people accredited with congenital word-blindness learning to read departs from the literature drastically, as, unlike all the previous articles that have been discussed, he argues it to be a difficult and (from the tone of his language) perhaps an impossible or even unnecessary endeavour. The differences between Rutherford's version of the diagnosis and that of the British ophthalmologists are perhaps indicative of the differences of the bio-politics in the USA and the UK. While eugenic movements were of considerable influence in both countries, negative eugenics became associated with the former and positive eugenics with the latter (Hansen and King, 2001: 244–5; Hasian, 1996: 21). For instance, eugenic policies such as sterilisation and eugenic immigration policies were only deployed in the USA during the first two decades of the twentieth century and not in the UK (Hansen and King 2001: 240).

Rutherford's description of how memory works in a child accredited as being congenitally word-blind is intriguing, in particular the allusion made by Rutherford to Impressionist painting, implying that memories in children accredited as being congenitally word-blind are distorted versions of reality. This description serves to further Rutherford's claims that children accredited with congenital word-blindness have malfunctioning brains. The description being articulated by Rutherford positions these subjects as somewhat less than human. Rutherford's diagnosis of dyslexia congenita would operate quite differently from congenital word-blindness. Seemingly not concerned with marking bodies in which the skills and attributes necessary to become economically productive *could* be fostered, Rutherford instead marked these bodies as waste. Rutherford's negative description of the characteristics that congenital word-blindness describes is related to the dominance of negative eugenics within the USA.

Defending the Borders

Hinshelwood's attempts to maintain a limited and specific version of the diagnosis he had been propagating (1895: 1565) should be understood as an attempt to maintain authority over the diagnosis. This preservation of a precise definition should be understood as an attempt to abate the funnel effect of the diagnosis being used to describe cases of increasingly less severe symptoms. With this having the effect of reducing the potency of the function that Hinshelwood's diagnosis performs—revealing a group of highly intelligent children amongst those considered backward and defective. Maintaining strict criteria for the diagnosis guarantees that it continues to have a precise function over a specifically defined population.

While not the originator of the diagnosis, Hinshelwood nevertheless attains a position, at least within the UK, where he is *the* authority on congenital word-blindness.[6] The conception of the diagnosis that he has engineered is a narrow one, with specific criteria and levels of attributes (1907: 1231) that must be reached to establish whether or not they are 'deserving' (1896: 1508), and therefore warrant the diagnosis 'congenital word-blindness'. A funnel effect seems to have taken place over the following years, with the diagnosis being attached to a wider group of people than Hinshelwood had envisioned (cases where the symptoms are not as pronounced as Hinshelwood maintained were necessary) and with the possibility of less severe cases being suggested in medical writing (Nettleship, 1901). In this light Hinshelwood offers the category of 'pure congenital word-blindness' as a way of maintaining and defending his vision:

> I use the term 'pure word-blindness'—that is, cases in which the brain of the patient is otherwise normal, and hence the intelligence and general mental powers of the patient good. Such cases must always be clearly distinguished from those-in which inability to learn to read is accompanied by a general lack of intelligence and general failure of all the mental powers. In such cases the difficulty in learning to read is not due to a purely local condition, but to a general lack of cerebral development, and hence are not included in the hopeful statement made about pure cases of. congenital word-blindness. (1907: 1232)

The introduction of 'pure word-blindness' is an important development, as Hinshelwood seems to be conceding that he can no longer exert control over who the diagnosis congenital of word-blindness applies to. As such, he attempts to defend the function that his diagnosis had hitherto served—to distinguish a group of extremely intelligent children who have an isolated difficulty in reading from the larger category of backward and defective children. Hinshelwood's concern with maintaining the potency of this operation results in the refinement of his own terminological machinery. The necessity of distinguishing between those children who would fit the diagnosis 'pure word-blindness' from the those who were now being diagnosed as congenitally word-blind would appear to be the same drive that concerned Hinshelwood in his earlier work in distinguishing children with congenital word-blindness from children accredited as being backward or defective (1900a, 1902). A particular group of children were seen as at risk of being misunderstood. Therefore, the diagnosis 'pure word-blindness' serves as the best tool to stop this from occurring. It is from this position that Hinshelwood refines his terminological device, so that these children can be further protected from unfair treatment as less severe cases begin to be diagnosed. Distinguishing between this group of children who, as the many cases recounted thus far (Hinshelwood, 1902, 1904, 1907; Nettleship, 1901; Thomas, 1905) have shown, are often exceptionally intelligent in other areas apart from reading, from those accredited as being backward or defective is the main function of the diagnosis for Hinshelwood. His goal is to maintain the potency of this function. Congenital word-blindness operates to refine those bodies who have been deemed uneducable, making this population smaller by marking some bodies as teachable if the correct technologies are deployed.

Conclusion

Considering the operation of a diagnosis such as congenital word-blindness within a bio-political analytical framework draws attention to the role diagnosis played in the reconfiguring of how parts of the population could be conceived of, organised and acted upon. This framework encourages the analysis of how a diagnosis operated to establish circuits through which power could flow, and how capillaries were instituted with other forms of diagnosis, as well as political and social programmes. 'Congenital word-blindness' functioned, as most medical categories do, by segmenting a population into smaller groups with shared characteristics. It served to foster the perception that a group with a shared set of characteristics could be more precisely directed, managed and cultivated. It identified a population previously considered to be backward, defective or feeble-minded, who were deemed to be uneducable, to, in fact, be teachable if the correct techniques were applied to their bodies. The diagnosis has thus been examined as a single technology in a larger machinery of government, concerned with proliferating desirable characteristics throughout the social body, through working in assemblage with the schooling system.

The first function that had to be achieved by the diagnosis was to establish that bodies marked with congenital word-blindness were not normal. This was achieved by establishing their difficulty in reading as localised. This was ascertained by measuring the different educational attributes of an individual and comparing this to the averages found in their peer groups. By working in assemblage with the norm, congenital word-blindness was able to generalise relations of power that were concerned with the individual body to the body of the population (Ewald, 1990, 1991). The process of differentiation was, however, taking place in relation to two poles, as the diagnosis also served to distinguish the

bodies in question from the category backward or defective. The localisation of the defective attribute isolated to a single part of the brain,
rather than being a general difficulty with learning, marked bodies as
distinct from both those bodies accredited as normal, and backward
or defective. Being diagnosed with congenital word-blindness marked
the individual as being closer to the normal body, rather then being
understood as backward, defective or feeble-minded because there was
considerable hope that, albeit with the right intervention, a successful
career could be achieved (Nettleship, 1901: 64).

The marking of these bodies as having the potential to become normal allowed the writers to make strong cases as to why specialist educational programmes should be developed to foster the development of
these children. The potential economic productivity of these individuals marked their localised difficulties with reading as a deserving defect
(Davis, 1995). An individual diagnosed with congenital word-blindness
could *become* an economically productive individual. The numerous
accounts are provided by the writers of cases of children accredited with
word-blindness achieving successful careers, despite their specific difficulties (Nettleship, 1901: 64). The narratives recounted of the children
in question, utilising their general intelligence to disguise their specific
difficulties, all gave weight to the development of these programmes.
The successes in educating some of these children, and the specificity of
their difficulties, distinguished these children from those accredited as
backward, defective or feeble-minded, and imbued the diagnosis with
a moral gloss, which is in some of texts quite pronounced (Hinshelwood, 1902). The version of congenital word-blindness propagated by
Hinshelwood and Thomas should be considered as a specific technology through which a strategy of government concerned with proliferating literacy throughout the population was enacted. Hinshelwood
(1896, 1902, 1904, 1907) and Thomas (1905) were attempting to assem-
ble a machinery of government, that would examine all backward and
defective children, sifting through this population, searching for individuals whose difficulties were localised to reading, segregating them
from the mainstream educational population and applying specialised
techniques to them.

While Hinshelwood's blueprint of the diagnosis was broadly accepted
within the UK, in the USA challenges were presented to his clinical
assumptions. Jackson (1905) presented a challenge to Hinshelwood's
dominance over reading difficulties by questioning the terminology
associated with the diagnosis and inserting a different aetiological
component into the diagnostic device. Rutherford's (1909) adaptation

of the hereditary hypothesis, first proposed by Thomas (1905), took the diagnosis into unchartered political territory, recalibrating the hereditary element of the diagnosis and aligning it with eugenic political concerns. Rutherford's (1909) differing views on the diagnosis, and his alternative terminology, are seemingly derived from his political positions. His politics are distinctly different to those we find in the language of British ophthalmologists, and his language and rhetoric would sit happily amongst those of the eugenicists of the day. The diagnosis here operates to show how a family history that is considered to be defective leads to various characteristics being passed down from one generation to the next, and are accredited as problems or defects. Dyslexia congenita is established as being related to various undesirable conditions and is ultimately conceived of as a reversion to a pre-civilised type, resulting from 'defective hereditary material' (Rutherford, 1909: 487). To be accredited with this diagnosis would, therefore, carry negative connotations.

In the USA and in the UK there were different logics underpinning the eugenic movements. In the USA the movement gained more influence on policy than in the first decades of the twentieth century, with eugenic immigration and sterilisation policies established. Policies of this type did not have equivalents in the UK (Hasian, 1996), which therefore produced two movements with quite different characters. Eugenics in the USA had a disposition that has been referred to as negative eugenics, while eugenics in the UK had a character that has been referred to as positive. The different character of the eugenic movements in the two countries was related to the formation of the make-up of bio-politics in each country. In turn, this was related to interactions with their different eugenic movements. The different variants of the diagnosis produced in either country seem to reflect the differing styles of bio-politics that were prevailing in these regions. The operations that these different versions of diagnosis performed were distinct. Rutherford's (1909) and Hinshewlood's versions of congenital word-blindness imbued very different moral values onto the bodies that they diagnosed. While the British ophthalmologists had a relatively unified position, internationally ophthalmologists were split fighting over the jurisdiction in various ways. This perhaps weakened their jurisdiction over congenital reading difficulties, opening the possibility for other disciplines to establish a jurisdiction over the diagnosis. I will explore this question in the following chapters.

Throughout this chapter I have tried to show how congenital word-blindness operated as a technology of power and how the function of this technology changed when the diagnosis was recalibrated through, for example, the insertion of a new aetiology. I have identified how North American challenges to Hinshelwood concentrated their criticisms on the terminology around the diagnosis, its aetiological components leading it to perform similar operations, but, in the case of Rutherford, being associated with a very different strategy of government. A minor recalibration of a technology of power allows it to operate with an array of different machineries of government, and be deployed to achieve the goals and strategies of government that it may have hitherto seemed incompatible with.

6
Psychological Explanations of Congenital Word-blindness

During the final years of the nineteenth century and the early years of the twentieth century the only discipline concerned with congenital reading difficulties was ophthalmology. This monopoly changed near the end of the first decade of the twentieth century when Lightner Witmer placed reading difficulties at the centre of the discipline of clinical psychology that he was attempting to establish. Over the course of the next two decades, reading difficulties were several times the subject of articles in *The Psychological Clinic*, and, later, congenital word-blindness became a specific area of research for those associated with the journal. The way the operation, fashioned by psychologists, differed from the ophthalmologists will be detailed in this chapter. To account for psychology's growing jurisdiction over reading difficulties, the relationship between psychology and education during this period will be explored.

Clinical psychology is often considered to be a forerunner of school psychology (Compas and Gotlib, 2002). Witmar has been elevated to the position of the founder of clinical psychology by most historians of this discipline. Witmar studied under Wilhelm Wundt in Germany and returned to the USA to replace his former teacher, James Cattel, as head of the psychology laboratory at the University of Pennsylvania (Compas and Gotlib, 2002). Witmer was concerned with the transformation of psychological knowledge into practices that could be applied to bodies to proliferate or augment desirable characteristics or attributes. Witmer (1896, 1897) had been studying methods by which psychological expertise could be deployed in non-clinical settings, and this provides an explanation for his interest in educational concerns. Upon taking over Cattel's laboratory in 1896, Witmer re-directed the laboratory's focus, establishing the psychological clinic (Compas and Gotlib, 2002). The clinic was concerned with applying psychological knowledge to the practical purpose of improving the educational performance of children considered to be difficult. A detailed exposition of Witmer's goals for the clinic, and his vision for psychology is given below as a means of establishing the horizon in which his (and those who published in his journal) version of the diagnosis was formed. Witmer's clinic at the University of Pennsylvania and the founding of *The Psychological Clinic*, constituted a space around which various disparate interests were able to coalesce and eventually ossify into educational psychology. This was in a similar fashion to how Sydney Stephenson's journal, *Ophthalmoscope*, provided a central axis upon which ophthalmologists could focus their attentions concerning congenital word-blindness (as described in Chapters 4 and 5). *The Psychological Clinic* provided an outlet for psychologists to publish articles concerned with word-blindness and many related, yet tangential, areas, and have them directed towards the main stream of the discipline. By providing a location at the centre of the discipline for psychological research concerned with congenital readings difficulties, *The Psychological Clinic* considered congenital reading as a central problematic of clinical psychology.

The discipline of clinical psychology was concerned with the practical applicability of knowledge (Witmer, 1907a: 4). It was concerned with training psychological experts for schools, and made a concerted effort to establish links with schools, hospital schools and schools for those children accredited as feeble-minded (Wimter, 1907a: 4). The direct concern with establishing these relations meant that it was part of the discipline's focus to institutionalise itself, to become embedded in the practices of teachers and other professionals, rather than being a secondary concern to the research, as it had been to the British ophthalmologists. This, no doubt, made the institutionalisation of the rationales and vocabularies of this discipline more successful than competing assemblages. In fact, it was precisely because of this focus that the conception of reading difficulties associated with *The Psychological Clinic* was able to gain institutional acceptance in non-psychological sites.

Historically, Witmer's importance to the formation of the discipline (Compas and Gotlib, 2002) and his editorship of *The Psychological Clinic*, combined with the interest in reading difficulties, propelled the diagnosis from being a concern of ophthalmology, in centripetal fashion, towards the centre of the emergent discipline of clinical psychology. The diagnosis made this movement at a significant point in history, which saw the rise of the modern psychology of the individual as it has become to be known to us today. It was at this point that it attained its structure, and its influence upon other fields augmented (Rose, 1984). Nikolas Rose (1985: 199) has argued that a focus on the child is instrumental for the formation of the psychology of the individual. *The Psychological Clinic* evidences this, as various articles were concerned with problematics such as school reports (Volkman and Noble, 1915), feeble-minded children (Witmer, 1913), gifted children (Witmer, 1919) and intelligence tests (Witmer, 1922). It has been argued that clinical psychology is the forerunner to the discipline of school psychology (Philips, 1990: 7). A regular discussion of congenital reading difficulties within a journal whose concerns configured the anatomy of educational psychology, established amnesia visualis verbalis and, later, congenital reading difficulties as a diagnostic to be deployed by educational psychologists. I will now describe how psychology began to gain dominance over ophthalmology in this field.

The Objectives of *The Psychological Clinic*

In the first issue of *The Psychological Clinic* Witmer published an account of his vision of clinical psychology (1907a). This manifesto of sorts utilised two case studies: one analogous to congenital word-blindness, the other to acquired word-blindness. However, it be must noted that this terminology is not used and references to any of the aforementioned literature are not present. It was also the first paper on congenital reading difficulties to be published in a psychology journal; moreover, it was also the first article on the topic to be published by a psychologist. In his journal, Witmer was attempting to develop clinical psychology as a coherent subfield of the discipline. It is of note that reading difficulties of both the acquired and congenital form were present at the formation of this sub-discipline of psychology (Witmer, 1907a).

In the inaugural issue of *The Psychological Clinic* Witmer published an article describing how his psychological clinic had operated for the last decade (1907a). This account was given so that other psychologists could utilise this rationale and deploy it in their own practices. This paper necessitates a lengthy discussion, as the examples that Witmer uses to outline his vision of clinical psychology are two cases of what he terms 'visual deafness', a diagnosis that symptomatically seems to be essentially analogous to word-blindness. The centrality of reading difficulties to Witmer's clinic, the journal and the emergent sub-discipline can be deduced from its place of exposition in this article.

Witmer's psychological clinic operated at the University of Pennsylvania from 1897 (Compas and Gotlib, 2002; Witmer 1907a). Children from schools in Philadelphia and adjacent cities were studied (Compas and Gotlib, 2002; Witmer 1907a). These children had made themselves conspicuous to either their teachers or parents 'because of an inability to progress in school work as rapidly as other children, or because of moral defects which rendered them difficult to manage under ordinary discipline' (Witmer, 1907a: 1). Witmer's concern was to study problematised children who were considered to be difficult, rather than impossible, to educate. The distinction here is paramount, as it was believed that study and experimentation would lead to the development of an array of rigorous methods and technologies that would allow for an improvement in these children's educational performances (Witmer, 1907a: 4).

The agenda for *The Psychological Clinic* was to foster a better understanding of difficult children, and develop methods to sort, diagnose and educate them. Witmer outlined his principles for practical work in psychology (*The Psychological Clinic* being part of this project) in his 1896 address to the American Psychological Association. He then reproduced these principles in his outline of the clinic's purpose (they were then reprinted in the inaugural issue of the journal):

- The investigation of the phenomena of mental development in school children, as manifested more particularly in mental and moral retardation, by means of the statistical and clinical methods.
- A psychological clinic, supplemented by a training school in the nature of a hospital school, for the treatment of all classes of children suffering from retardation or physical defects interfering with school progress.
- The offering of practical work to those engaged in the professions of teaching and medicine, and to those interested in social work, in the observation and training of normal and retarded children.
- The training of students for a new profession—that of the psychological expert, who should find his career in connection with the school system, through the examination and treatment of mentally and morally retarded children, or in connection with the practice of medicine.

(1907a: 4)

Psychology, for Witmer, needed to establish links with institutions such as schools, provide expertise to teachers, physicians and social workers, and develop a new professional neologism, 'the psychological expert'. The psychological expert would become necessary to the school system through engaging in the examination and treatment of children accredited as mentally and morally retarded with the remit to improve their education attainment. The psychological expert was set to become an important part of the machinery of government concerned with fostering the development of as many bodies as possible in schools. The psychologist would form part of a machinery of government devoted to the task of educating bodies previously considered inhospitable to educational techniques. This plan to diffuse psychological expertise throughout institutions and professions was concerned with producing and cultivating populations; making psychological knowledge indispensable to their operations would augment the institutionalization of Witmer's conception of the discipline, thus allowing for psychological practices to be applied to new sites through these emergent capillaries. This diffusion of psychological expertise was, of course, taking place amongst a wider distribution of expertise and authority that Rose (1993) argues characterises a liberal style of bio-political governing. The successful institutionalisation of psychology helped to solidify certain diagnoses, such as congenital reading difficulties, as being under a psychological auspice. Owing to the emphasis that Witmer placed on the practical applicability of psychological knowledge, his diagnostic catgories were likely to proliferate among a wider field of experts. Witmer was certainly more concerned with establishing links with schools and other disciplines than Hinshelwood appeared to be.

The Psychological Clinic's principle concern was the education of children whose schooling was understood to be suffering because of either an accredited physical defect or so-called retardation (Witmer, 1907a: 4). This positioned the discipline in an advantageous position to develop and maintain a firm jurisdiction of all manner of educational difficulties including those with reading. It will be argued hereafter that the psychological clinics (and psychology more generally) were more successful in establishing links with educationalists. This was an important factor in the jurisdiction over the diagnosis moving from ophthalmology to psychology. It is also noteworthy that there appeared to be quite a different trajectory developing in the USA and in the UK. Congenital reading difficulties had been established as being under the remit of ophthalmologists in the UK; however, in the USA, the jurisdiction over reading difficulties had been formed by clinical psychologists. The imperialistic rationale of clinical psychologists desired to actively foster connections with schools and educationalists. This is one way of accounting for the decline of ophthalmology's slipping jurisdiction over reading difficulties and the rise of psychology's jurisdiction.

The psychological clinic utilised medical examinations to generate a full picture of the child in question. It was deployed as a diagrammatic device. Specific physical tests were deployed as part of the examination assemblage; psychological diagnosis could then be made with confidence and assurance that no medical condition was interfering with the subjects' intellectual faculties. The examination, as deployed by the psychological clinic, utilised the technologies of these two disciplines in assemblage, both deployed onto the body being studied:

> When brought to the psychological clinic, such children are given a physical and mental examination; if the result of this examination shows it to be desirable, they are then sent to specialists for the eye or ear, for the nose and throat, and for nervous diseases, one or all, as each case may require. The result of this conjoint medical and psychological examination is a diagnosis of the child's mental and physical condition and the recommendation of appropriate medical and pedagogical treatment. The progress of some of these children has been followed for a term of years. (Witmer, 1907a: 1)

The Psychological Clinic's goal of studying and developing methods for describing, segmenting and training children whose education was thought to be difficult made the journal a likely site for congenital reading difficulties to be discussed. Witmer's clinic hoped to recommend the appropriate medical and pedagogical treatment on a case-by-case basis.

As a way of illustrating how the University of Pennsylvania's psychological clinic operated, Witmer chooses to recount two cases. The first is a condition seemingly analogous to acquired word-blindness, and the second is comparable to congenital word-blindness. The use of these cases illustrates to the reader how the University of Pennsylvania's psychological clinic operated, displaying how reading difficulties, whether they be in their acquired or congenital forms, were one of the central concerns of this emergent sub-discipline of psychology from its conception. Witmer describes how the boy at the centre of his study was sent to see various experts, oculists and neurologists on the recommendation of the Superintendent of Schools, giving evidence of the link between Philadelphia schools and the psychological clinic. This is in contrast to many of the ophthalmological writers, who came into contact with the patients by their parents bringing them to see an eye specialist (Hinshelwood, 1902: 94–5, 1907: 1230). *The Psychological Clinic's* attempts to forge links with the educational system meant that it had a wider access to bodies than the British ophthalmologists. The operation of Witmer's clinic shows some of the methods it deployed to access populations:

> To illustrate the operation of the psychological clinic, take a recent case sent to the laboratory from a city of Pennsylvania, not far from

Philadelphia. The child was brought by his parents, on the recommendation of the Superintendent of Schools. Examination revealed a boy ten years of age, without apparent physical defect, who had spent four years at school, but had made so little progress that his ignorance of the printed symbols of the alphabet made it necessary to use the illiterate card to test his vision. Nothing in the child's heredity or early history revealed any ground for the suspicion of degeneracy, nor did the child's physical appearance warrant this diagnosis. The boy appeared to be of normal intelligence, except for the retardation in school work. The examination of the neurologist to whom he was sent, Dr. William G. Spiller, confirmed the absence of conspicuous mental degeneracy and of physical defect. The oculist, Dr. William C. Posey, found nothing more serious than a slight far-sighted astigmatism, and the examination of Dr. George C. Stout for adenoids, gave the child a clean bill of health, so far as the nose and pharynx were concerned. On the conclusion of this examination he was, necessarily, returned to the school from which he came, with the recommendation to the teacher of a course of treatment to develop the child's intelligence. It will require at least three months' observation to determine whether his present pedagogical retardation is based upon an arrest of cerebral development or is merely the result of inadequate methods of education. This case is unequivocally one for the psychologist. (1907a: 1–2)

The development of a course of treatment to improve the child's intelligence is something that Hinshelwood (1902, 1907) and the ophthalmological writers (Thomas, 1905) had advocated (see Chapter 5). It was, however, only in Hinshelwood's final article on the subject that he turned explicitly to this task (Hinshelwood, 1912). The positing of inadequate educational methods as a reason for the child's difficulty has not been proposed in the literature thus far discussed; the time frame of 3 months that Witmer indicates as necessary to exclude this possibility and confidently make a diagnosis based upon a specific educational difficulty, is a newly inserted diagnostic criterion.

Witmer recounts how he first came into contact with this patient, whose difficulties with language were restricting him in his studies as a student at a preparatory college.

My attention was first drawn to the phenomena of retardation in the year 1889. At that time, while a student of psychology at the University of Pennsylvania, I had charge of the English branches in a college preparatory school of Philadelphia. In my classes at this academy I was called upon to give instruction in English to a boy preparing for entrance to college, who showed a remarkable deficiency in the English language. His compositions seldom contained a single sentence that had been correctly formed. For example, there was little or no distinction between the present and the past tenses of verbs; the endings of many words were clipped off, and this was especially noticeable in those words in which a final ending distinguished the plural from the singular, or an adverb from an adjective. As it seemed doubtful whether he would ever be able to enter college without special instruction in English, I was engaged to tutor him in the English branches. (1907a: 2)

This description of the boy's accredited problems underlies the specific, yet pronounced, difficulties that hampered his overall academic performance. A comparison can be drawn to the cases encountered in earlier chapters by the British ophthalmologists, owing to the specificity of the subjects' difficulties. They differ, however, as Witmer does not so strongly try to emphasise the subject's intelligence through anecdote and a strong use of language in the same manner as Hinshelwood (1896) and Thomas (1905) had. The aetiology of the subject's specific difficulty is described, with an emphasis on the articulation of words—a diagnostic factor that had hitherto been absent from the ophthalmological writings. Witmer is again adding diagnostic criteria—a new component to the technology:

I had no sooner undertaken this work than I saw the necessity of beginning with the elements of language and teaching him as one would teach a boy, say, in the third grade. Before long I discovered that I must start still further back. I had found it impossible, through oral and written exercises, to fix in his mind the elementary forms of words as parts of speech in a sentence. This seemed to be owing to the fact that he had verbal deafness. He was quite able to hear even a faint sound, like the ticking of a watch, but he could not hear the difference in the sound of such words as *grasp* and *grasped*. This verbal deafness was associated with, and I now believe was probably caused by, a defect of articulation. Thus the boy's written language was a fairly exact replica of his spoken language; and he probably heard the words that others spoke as he himself spoke them. I therefore undertook to give him an elementary training in articulation to remedy the defects which are ordinarily corrected, through imitation, by the time a child is three or four years old. I gave practically no attention to the subjects required in English for college entrance, spending all my time on the drill in articulation and in perfecting his verbal audition and teaching him the simplest elements of written language. The result was a great improvement in all his written work, and he succeeded in entering the college department of the University of Pennsylvania in the following year. (1907a: 2)

The introduction of the diagnosis 'verbal deafness', without reference to the various terminological devices that have been deployed to portray the symptoms that Witmer describes, shows either a lack of knowledge, or a disinterest in the debates and research that had already existed around reading difficulties. 'Verbal deafness' is a curious coinage, not seen before or again in the literature; while being symptomatically analogous to word-blindness, it sounds almost like its antonym.

The same boy was encountered again by Witmer some years later when he was teaching at the University of Pennsylvania. It is noted that he had been able to progress though his college education, but recounted that his deficiencies in language resulted in him failing in the final year:

In 1894–95, I found him as a college student in my classes at the University of Pennsylvania. His articulation, his written discourse and his verbal audition were very deficient for a boy of his years. In consequence he was unable to acquire the technical terminology of my branch, and I have no doubt that he passed very few examinations excepting through the sympathy of his instructors who overlooked the serious imperfections of his written work, owing to the fact that he was in other respects a fair student. When it came to the final examinations for the bachelor's degree, however, he failed and was compelled to repeat much of the work of his senior year. He subsequently entered and graduated from one of the professional departments of the University. His deficiencies in language, I believe, have never been entirely overcome. (1907a: 2–3)

It is assumed that the subject passed examinations on account of the sympathies of teaching staff, which, in Witmer's view, overlooked the problems with his written work. The difficulties in acquiring the professional vocabulary required by Witmer's department are detailed in conjunction with the difficulties he had in passing his final exams. The student transferred to one of the professional branches of the university where he completed his studies. With the student never overcoming his difficulties with language, a less favourable picture of the curability of children accredited with congenital reading difficulties is formed (Hinshelwood, 1912; Nettleship, 1901).

Witmer underlines the importance of beginning the training of the subject as early as possible, an emphasis previously found in Hinshelwood (Hinshelwood, 1896: 1508). Witmer accounts for the failure in improvement to be the result of the treatment not beginning at an early enough point in the boy's life:

> I felt very keenly how much this boy was losing through his speech defect. His school work, his college course, and doubtless his professional career were all seriously hampered. I was confident at the time, and this confidence has been justified by subsequent experience with similar cases, that if he had been given adequate instruction in articulation in the early years of childhood, he could have overcome his defect. With the improvement in articulation there would have come an improved power of apprehending spoken and written language. That nothing was done for him in the early years, nor indeed at any time, excepting for the brief period of private instruction in English and some lessons in elocution, is remarkable, for the speech defect was primarily owing to an injury to the head in the second year of life, and his father was a physician who might have been expected to appreciate the necessity of special training in a case of retardation caused by a brain injury. (1907a: 3)

No description of how the subject acquired the injury is given, revealing a distinctly different focus to the cases of acquired word-blindness discussed in Chapter 4 (Broadbent, 1872; Hinshelwood, 1895) where the injury is described in detail, often with descriptions of what specific region of the brain had been affected by the injury. Witmer spent considerably more time than the ophthalmological writers detailing how the subject should be taught since acquiring a difficulty with reading (Hinshelwood, 1895, 1896, 1900a; Morgan, 1896; Thomas, 1905). The Psychological Clinic's emphasis upon training and making knowledge applicable to various experts and practical situations should be considered an important factor in the success of psychology establishing a jurisdiction over specific reading difficulties. Rather than being a tangential concern, developing practices to teach and train children diagnosed with a reading difficultly was central to their research.

Witmer continues by outlining the rationale of clinical psychology with his description of a second case. This boy is initially described as a chronically bad speller. The following description of this case is comparable to descriptions of congenital word-blindness:

> The second case to attract my interest was a boy fourteen years of age, who was brought to the laboratory of psychology by his grade teacher. He was one of those children of great interest to the teacher, known to the profession as a chronic bad speller. His teacher, Miss Margaret T. Maguire, now the supervising principal of a grammar school of Philadelphia, was at that time a student of psychology at the University of Pennsylvania; she was imbued with the idea that a psychologist should be able, through examination, to ascertain the causes of a deficiency in spelling and to recommend the appropriate pedagogical treatment for its amelioration or cure. (1907a: 3)

This subject came to Witmer's attention because of the actions of a teacher who was committed to the notion that psychologists should be able to offer an appropriate plan for pedagogical treatment. Witmer described how he had, at this time, found no studies in psychology that were concerned with the treatment of a deficiency in spelling. Hinshelwood understood congenital word-blindness as a deficiency in memory, and Witmer made a similar diagnosis for this case:

> With this case, in March, 1896, the work of the psychological clinic was begun. At that time I could not find that the science of psychology had ever addressed itself to the ascertainment of the causes and treatment of a deficiency in spelling. Yet here was a simple developmental defect of memory; and memory is a mental process of which the science of psychology is supposed to furnish the only authoritative knowledge. It appeared to me that if psychology was worth anything to me or to others it should be able to assist the efforts of a teacher in a retarded case of this kind. (1907a: 3)

The worth of the discipline of psychology is called into question for Witmer unless it can offer practical techniques for teaching children with specific difficulties. This again restates how his vision of psychology was concerned with the development of practical knowledge that could be deployed in the cultivation of children who presented problem for their teachers. Witmer describes how he worked with these children, developing his methods with little or no precedents in the history of psychology:

> The absence of any principles to guide me made it necessary to apply myself directly to the study of these children, working out my methods as I went along. In the spring of 1896 I saw several other cases of children suffering from the retardation of some special function, like that of spelling, or from general retardation, and I undertook the training of these children for a certain number of hours each week. Since that time the psychological clinic has been regularly conducted in connection with the laboratory of psychology at the University of Pennsylvania. The study of these cases has also formed a regular part of the instruction offered to students in child psychology. (1907a: 4)

The psychological clinic at the University of Pennsylvania and the associated journal had two declared objects of knowledge: children accredited with specific difficulties and children accredited with general retardation. This suggests that the process of differentiation between these two groups that Hinshelwood had been keen to establish in his research was less emphasised at the psychological clinic (Witmer, 1907a: 1). Studying children with specific difficulties became a part of the general education of students enrolled in child psychology at the University of Pennsylvania (Witmer, 1907a). Witmer's position allowed him to influence a generation of psychologists focusing their training upon the practical applicability of psychology, and establishing children accredited as defective as the main object of clinical psychology's investigation. The development of a disciplinary focus, and Witmer's position as educator, allowed for the dissipation of this rationale throughout the academic field and many professional or practical fields that his students became involved in. For graduates of the University of Pennsylvania's psychology programme, the study of children accredited as defective was a cornerstone of psychology; children with specific reading difficulties were understood as one type of defective that could be studied. The investigation of similar conditions on both sides of the Atlantic concurrently may, of course, just have been a coincidence, but the possibility of emergent rationalities of government on both sides of the Atlantic, making conditions admissible to the development of these diagnoses, must be considered. The links that the University of Pennsylvania's psychological clinic made with schools and other educational institutions played a crucial role in fostering the psychologist's conception of the diagnosis to be disseminated through educational journals and into American schools. Psychology appears to have been better placed than ophthalmology to disperse its diagnosis into educational environments, as its technologies and practices were more amenable to this environment, therefore gaining access to a larger population.

Reading Difficulties in *The Psychological Clinic*

In the next issue of *The Psychological Clinic*, Witmer (1907b) published another paper concerned with a specific reading difficulty. The dominant clinical terminology (associated with ophthalmology) is again eschewed in favour of a term of Witmer's own coinage 'amnesia visualis verbalis'; his previous coinage of 'visual deafness' is therefore rejected. Rather than this interest in reading difficulties being understood as an attempt to wrestle the jurisdiction of a diagnosis from another discipline, it is perhaps more pertinent to see this as a small part of the larger project of formalising psychology as a discipline (Rose, 1984). The deployment of new terminological devices should be understood as a challenge to the conceptual, clinical and practical rationales associated with the particular discipline of ophthalmology. The characteristics that amnesia visualis verbalis describes are considered by Witmer to be firmly under the auspice of psychology as opposed to ophthalmology. With a new terminological formulation, in this case amnesia visualis verbalis, comes new moral, political and scientific values. The technology may depend upon different values, and be amenable to a different political rationale or be dependent upon a particular strategy of government. The positioning of amnesia visualis verbalis within such a framework shall now be explored

Amnesia visualis verbalis avoids many of the previous terminological formulations, or, indeed, terminological components utilised to develop a diagnostic category for specific reading difficulties. The deployment of amnesia, rather than blindness, situates the diagnosis as associated with memory rather than sight, inscribing the diagnosis firmly onto the brain, and therefore weakening the connection with the ophthalmologists. Congenital reading difficulties are being placed firmly under the jurisdiction of psychology. This is, of course, a key development, as memory had continued to be the focus since Broadbent (1872). However, the suffix blindness was still widely deployed, despite criticism from both the physicians involved in articulating congenital word-blindness and those who suggested alternative diagnostic categories (Clairborne, 1906; Rutherford, 1909; Wernickle in Claiborne, 1906; Wernickle in

Hinshelwood 1904). In this case, memory is an attribute that falls under the authority of psychologists, and as the psychology of the individual continued to develop (Rose, 1984, 1999), the logic of specific difficulties concerned with an aspect of memory falling under the jurisdiction of psychology would intensify. While Witmer eschews formulations such as congenital word-blindness (Hinshelwood, 1900a; Morgan, 1896) and dyslexia congenita (Rutherford, 1909) in favour of his own formulation for the explanation of its specific characteristics he is describing—amnesia visualis verbalis—this is then framed as being one of many congenital aphasias (that were, indeed, studied in the pages of *The Psychological Clinic*). The positioning of reading difficulties in part of a group of an interrelated array of diagnostic categories—congenital aphasias, which clinical psychology has a jurisdiction over—illustrates that related diagnoses are being deployed in assemblage with amnesia visualis verbalis to help develop a jurisdiction over congenital reading difficulties for psychology. The group of diagnoses, amnesia visulais verbalis, is considered to be related to a diagnosis that Broadbent (1872) describes, as they were thought to be difficulties with particular and localised intellectual attributes.

Witmer's comparison of amnesia visualis verbalis to other congenital aphasias shows an awareness that research has already been carried out in the area. This suggests that he was deliberately ignoring the vast amount of literature already written about this topic. The very prominent location of some of these articles in *The Lancet* and the *British Medical Journal* would suggest that if Witmer had a serious clinical interest in congenital aphasia he would be familiar with at least some of these writers. Witmer advances a non-pathological understanding of specific reading difficulties and other specific aphasias he is interested in. Witmer argued that:

> While it is doubtless true that brain injuries may produce aphasia and amusia in children and if such injuries occur during uterine life the condition may properly be described as congenital, nevertheless I believe we must consider that congenital aphasia and amusia do not rest upon a pathological condition of the brain, but are indicative of a tendency to biological variation appearing in the affected children restrictedly as variation of the functional activities of language and music. Congenital aphasia and amusia are to be explained in biological terms, in somewhat the same manner as we should undertake to explain left-handedness in about 2 per cent of the race. (1907b)

In the same mode as Hinshelwood (1912), Witmer wishes to assert the developmental character of congenital aphasia, against the hypothesis that congenital aphasia and amusia may actually be acquired aphasias gained during birth or in very early life. It is crucial here to note that Witmer is positing congenital apahsia and amusia to be the result of variance within the functional activities of language and music, comparing them with left-handedness, rather than considering them as pathological. Congenital aphasia is understood here as a 'tendency to biological variation' and not a 'pathological condition of the brain'. This rhetoric, to some degree, achieves the naturalising or normalising of the variation. It is removed from being associated with pathologies. Of course, this clinical distinction embedded moral values as those accredited as having a congenital aphasia are considered not that different to the norm, and should subsequently be treated in a similar way. Positioning the characteristics he was describing as non-pathological should be understood as necessary owing to the American eugenics movement's influence on how pathological characteristics should be treated. Witmer's version of a diagnosis dealing with congenital reading difficulties performs a very different operation to that of his countryman, Rutherford (1909). Like Hinshelwood (1896, 1900a, 1902) before him, Witmer was concerned with emphasising that those accredited with congenital aphasia should not be considered to be defective. The specific diagnostic category of each congenital aphasia would therefore operate as a technology of power to mark a body as having a 'tendency to biological variation' (Witmer, 1907b), rather than being understood as backward, defective or feebleminded. They were, therefore, technologies of power concerned with enacting a very subtle and precise process of differentiation, removing the negative connotations of being considered backward or defective from a body, while establishing a significant enough difference to allow for specialist teaching techniques to be deployed.

Witmer's diagnostic apparatus performs a similar function to that of Hinshelwood's (1896, 1900a, 1902) in distinguishing between those cases of word-blindness where other cerebral skills could be invoked to improve the subject's difficulties with language, and those who were accredited as having a more general failure of intelligence. In a time when having characteristics considered to be pathological was becoming increasingly problematic (owing to the rise of eugenics), the necessity of affirming a diagnostic group as having a 'tendency to biological variation' (Witmer, 1907b) was needed to fashion technologies that would allow these individuals to attain normality. Congenital aphasia operated in assemblage with the norm and other technologies of measurement, making the 'normal' and 'abnormal' operate as spectral categories that could be applied to specific attributes rather than absolute categories that described a person in their totality (this is similar to Hinshelwood, as discussed in Chapter 5). This increasingly complex machinery of government facilitated the flow of power onto the body in a microscopic fashion, allowing for specific attributes to be cultivated in bodies and proliferated throughout the population.

Witmer (1907b) takes issue with explanations of congenital word-blindness that suggest it is engendered by a brain injury at birth, even though an earlier paper of his had suggested this as a possibility (Witmer, 1907a). Witmer (1907b) posits congenital aphasia and amusia to be the result of a variance within the functional activities of language and music, contrasting them with left-handedness, rather than considering them as pathological. The comparison here frames congenital word-blindness as an acceptable and relatively non-problematic difference, rather than a pathology. The construction of non-pathological difference is important in establishing those accredited with congenital aphasia as curable, but also as it gives the psychological clinic a vocation to improve the educational attainment of those children who have specific and localised learning difficulties resulting from discrepancies between various attributes in their intelligence. The University of Pennsylvania's psychological clinic was able to transform bodies previously accredited as pathological and problematic into non-problematic or less problematic bodies.

While Hinshelwood's conception of congenital word-blindness was still positioned within the field of aphasic disorders, the term aphasia itself had been increasingly absent from his post-1900 papers, suggesting an attempt to establish distance between congenital word-blindness and these aphasic categories. Discussions of reading difficulties in *The Psychological Clinic* firmly placed it as one among many congenital aphasias, eroding Hinshelwood's jurisdiction over the diagnosis by solidifying its connection to a family of diagnoses that were increasingly under the auspice of psychology. Town (1911), a researcher who also published in Witmer's *The Psychological Clinic*, like Witmer also situated specific reading difficulties in the context of the wider subject of acquired aphasias:

> There is probably no subject in the whole field of psychiatry which can boast a larger literature than aphasia. To read only the most important contributions since the publication of Broca's theory in 1861, would be an Herculean task. Nevertheless, one variety of the condition, its congenital form, has, in the heat of controversy been

much neglected. Many a man well versed in the literature of aphasia and practically conversant with its adult varieties is so unfamiliar with this conception of a congenital from that its mention arouses a smile and brings forth the query—'How can there be a loss of memory for language in any one or all of its forms, but this reasoning really contains a fallacy and the fallacy is a faulty conception of the meaning and scope memory'. (1911: 167)

Within the large field of studies of aphasias, congenital aphasias are described by Town as being a severely neglected area of research, full of many misunderstandings regarding the nature of memory. With aphasias being considered by the writers associated with *The Psychological Clinic* to be unquestionably under the auspice of psychology, the association of congenital word-blindness with ophthalmology in Britain appears to be an aberration, corrected by the growth in psychology's institutional importance. Acquired and congenital difficulties with language are described as being impairments regularly doubted even by experts on aphasia. These doubts partially explain why so many of the writers discussed thus far had been so concerned with defending the diagnosis against potential sceptics (Hinshelwood, 1907). As I have already argued (Chapters 4 and 5) severe cases were favoured as illustrative examples by researchers because they were less likely to be criticised by those who considered the diagnosis to be a questionable notion. The segmentation of intellectual attributes is continued as memory here is described as having two aspects—the ability to retain impressions and the ability to recall impressions:

> The process of memory is in reality a twofold one, it implies the ability to retrain impressions and the ability to recall them. These process are absolutely distinct, the first may be intact while recall is interfered with, though of course there can be no recall without an initial impressibility. (Town, 1911: 167)

The separation of these two functions allows for the conceptualisation of various types of congenital aphasia. Congenital reading difficulties are here being presented as a problem that results from a deficiency with one of these forms of memory. While this aetiology is similar to Hinshelwood (1896), the style of its expression and its association with psychology rather than ophthalmology, means that it should be counted as an aetiological innovation. The diagnosis has been recalibrated to operate as part of a different machinery of government.

Town's description of adults losing their language abilities owing to aphasia recalls Broadbent (1872) and Kussmaul's (1877) earlier papers on acquired word-blindness, and continues the theme of reconnecting congenital reading difficulties to aphasia that characterised Witmer's (1907a, 1907b) earlier work in *The Psychological Clinic*. The re-covering of similar ground suggests that the writers associated with *The Psychological Clinic* may have, indeed, been unaware of the work that the British ophthalmologists had conducted concerning a similar set of problems, but actively chose to ignore it so as to help establish their particular discipline. Town re-establishes the connection to acquired reading difficulties:

> In an adult who has much experience of language and formed a large vocabulary, aphasia betrays itself in an inability to understand or to recall or utter one familiar words; his daily occupation makes a constant demand upon his stock of already acquired verbal ideas, and little demand upon his ability to acquire news one, therefore his loss of power to recall is strikingly evident and his loss of impressibility remains unnoticed. (1911: 167)

The connection to acquired reading difficulties was less present in the ophthalmological papers reviewed in the preceding chapters, with most of the papers only having a cursory or, in some cases, no reference at all to acquired word-blindness. References to acquired word-blindness had, indeed, become less common as congenital word-blindness became a more established diagnosis (Hinshelwood, 1900a, 1900b, 1902, 1907; Nettleship, 1901; Thomas, 1905; Witmer, 1907b). Aphasia fell under the newly established domain of the psychology of the individual (Rose, 1984), with Town's (1911) restating of congenital reading difficulties as a form of aphasia perhaps moving it clearly under the jurisdiction of psychology. The need for the diagnostic category to perform the function of distinguishing children accredited with congenital reading difficulties from those accredited as feeble-minded is a theme that Town chooses to restate, much like Hinshelwood's (1896: 1508) conception of congenital word-blindness as being necessarily independent of any other mental defect:

> Aphasia then is an inability, total or partial, to understand or to use language in any one or all of its forms, such inability being independent of any other mental incapacity or of any deformity or disease affecting the organs of articulation. It is particularly necessary

to bear in mind those qualifications when considering the aphasias of childhood, as some authors writing of the feebleminded call all mute idiotic children who are not deaf aphasias, their standpoint being the exact opposite of that those mentioned above who are familiar with aphasias of adults. (1911: 168)

Establishing a difference between those with congenital reading difficulties and those accredited as feeble-minded is a more significant concern for Town (1911) than it was for Witmer (1907a, 1907b). A better understanding of this wide category—the feeble-minded—was advocated through its segmentation into various specific and localised difficulties. Clinical psychology aimed to create intravenous knowledge that could act upon subjects through the organisation of children accredited as feeble-minded into smaller categories, that is manageable units. This facilitated the deployment of methods to overcome their now better understood educational difficulties. Efforts could be directed away from those where there was little chance of improvement toward those children where a higher degree of improvement was likely after a modified educational programme had been installed.

A specific detail of how we can distinguish between a child that Town would consider to be an imbecile and a child with congenital aphasia is suggested. A study of the relation between the auditory and spoken vocabulary is stated as being indicative of the difference between the two populations:

In a normal child or an imbecile without special language defect, the auditory vocabulary always exceeds the spoken, but with this boy the opposite condition exists, and he gives no sign of understanding more then the following twelve words when spoken:

stocking	tooth	nose
dog	horse	mouth
baby	man	ears
bird	eyes	William

(Town, 1911: 176)

A discussion of a relation between spoken and auditory vocabularies is a diagnostic innovation, instituting a further way of distinguishing between the two populations. It recalls the first case that Witmer discussed (1907a) where he suggested that the subject's difficulties in articulation related to his specific reading difficulties. This relationship between reading, auditory and spoken vocabularies is seen as distinct during this period by the writers associated with *The Psychological Clinic*.

Town provides a description of a girl who he diagnosed as having a congenital difficulty with reading. The description of this girl illustrates that Town understood there to be a connection between what he dubbed bad hereditary and congenital aphasias, thus re-iterating some of the same themes that Rutherford (1909) had initiated:

> The little girl has a bad hereditary and her condition seems to be congenital. Her father, grandfather and one uncle drank heavily, and her father also uses tobacco to excess. Her parents were first cousins, and her mother was subjected to much worry and grief before the child's birth. She has had measles, whooping cough, mumps, chorea and otitis media, but never the slightest paralysis. She is a highly nervous child, unusually active and has splendid muscular control. She runs like a deer, and her history states that she climbs everywhere and loves to chase cattle. She uses her hands well, cuts well, and likes to scribble, using her left hand and producing remarkably regular lines of continuous scribe in imitation of a letter. (1911: 177)

The attributes that Town considers to be the girl's hereditary characteristics are listed. It is unclear whether the final aspects detailed by Town are to be considered as part of her bad hereditary or positive attributes. No references are made to the discussion of the character of congenital word-blindness in Thomas (1905), Hinshelwood (1907) or Stephenson (1907), providing further evidence that the writers associated with *The Psychological Clinic* could have been unaware of the ophthalmological literature on this subject or, alternatively, were attempting to distance themselves from it. In this discussion, a connection is instituted between what is dubbed bad hereditary and the child's congenital aphasia. While Town's tone is not as severe as Rutherford's (1909), it should be noted that both articles are written by Americans, illustrating that the American blueprint of the diagnostic category had a closer relation to eugenic themes than the category associated with Hinshelwood and the British ophthalmologists.

The next article on congenital aphasia, or congenital reading difficulties in *The Psychological Clinic* was, again, by Witmer (1916). Arthur, the boy who forms the case study of Witmer's (1916) 'Congenital Aphasia and Feeblemindedness—A Clinical Diagnosis', is described as being backward. This is a departure from Hinshelwood (1896, 1900a, 1902, 1907) and his associates (Nettleship, 1901; Thomas,

1905), who went to great lengths to expound the intelligence of the subjects they were describing to emphasise how these individuals could and should be distinguished from those accredited as lacking intelligence. Here, Witmer is less concerned with establishing a difference between these two groups than the ophthalmological writers, perhaps because the machinery of his discipline, psychology, could articulate relations of power in more specific directions and with a more forceful effect.

> I want to give you some facts. This boy, Arthur, is ten years and eight months old, nearly eleven years old. He told you he was in the second grade A, which is the first half of the second grade. Consequently he is backward in school progress. That is what we would call true backwardness, pedagogical backwardness. It is retardation on education scale. He is nearly eleven years old. He ought to be at least in the fourth grade, so that he shows two and perhaps we ought to say three years of backwardness. (1916: 184)

While Witmer does not break with describing his patients as backward in such a drastic fashion as Hinshelwood (1896, 1900a, 1902, 1907) by likening congenital verbal amnesia to being unable to sing a tune (a similar motif to his earlier comparison to left-handedness) it illustrates that he, too, is trying to distinguish between congenital aphasia and those accredited as feeble-minded, backward or defective. Witmer's descriptions illustrate that congenital aphasias are not to be seen as a significant barrier to educational attainment, thus establishing a crucial distinction between people diagnosed with congenital aphasias and those accredited as defective:

> Just as one boy hasn't got an ear for music, because he hasn't got the kind of brain that stores up musical tones, so this boy hasn't got the kind of brain which stores up memories of words and letters and sentences that are spoken to him. In his case it is probably a congenital verbal amnesia. (1916: 189)

Witmer presents children accredited with congenital verbal amnesia as having different types of brains rather than defective or malfunctioning brains. This theme was established in earlier papers in *The Psychological Clinic* (Town, 1911; Witmer, 1907b). Hinshelwood, in his book *Mind, Letter and Word-blindness* (1900b), and Kussmaul (1877) had already distinguished between various types of memory, suggesting that aphasias of various types are engendered by problems with the particular memory system, developing further the research of Broadbent (1872). Witmer restates (although it is not clear whether Witmer was aware of Hinshelwood or Kussmaul's research) this comparison by making the analogy with amusia, a parallel comparison he had outlined in his first paper on the subject (Witmer, 1907a):

> Are there any children born whom you can't teach to sing a tune? If so they would have amnesia musicalis, or amusia, a term applying to those who are tone-deaf and can't learn to sing. These others we can speak of as congenital illiterates, and since it has to do with language we may call it congenital aphasia. I would say this boy is probably not really feebleminded, but it looks as though he had congenital aphasia. (1916: 190)

Witmer does not deploy the term congenital word-blindness, seemingly preferring to refer to those considered to have a congenital difficulty with reading as 'congenital illiterates' or as having 'congenital aphasia'. Congenital word-blindness, the term associated with the British writers whose work was associated with the *Ophthalmoscope* is once again ignored (Hinshelwood, 1896, 1900a, 1902, 1907; Morgan, 1896; Nettleship, 1901; Thomas, 1905). Witmer repositions the diagnosis as part of an array of localised educational difficulties. Complex diagrams of human capabilities were thus forming as localised difficulties could be identified, assessed and measured. In the hands of the British ophthalmologists, congenital word-blindness had been established as distinct from aphasia. Witmer's terminological decision seems to re-emphasise the close relationship between congenital verbal amnesia and aphasia. Two reasons could be suggested for this re-emphasis upon aphasia: (1) that aphasia was a strong component of the psychologist's conceptual machinery, and it is thus unsurprising that Witmer (1907b, 1916) and Town (1911) both deployed these devices in their research owing to their familiarity with it; and (2) that these psychologists emphasised relations with an analogous diagnosis firmly within their jurisdiction, to make a claim for the diagnosis falling solely under the jurisdiction of their formalising discipline.

The earlier cases of congenital word-blindness focused upon pronounced examples. In some of the articles it was suggested that the diagnosis could only exist in profound cases (Hinshelwood, 1896: 1508, 1904). I argued in Chapter 5 that this privileging of accentuated examples of the characteristics that the diagnosis was concerned with was utilised for two main reasons: (1) to establish the diagnosis as a veritable diagnostic category less open to criticism; and (2) to allow the diagnosis' operation to be more potent, allowing the identified difference to be marked more intensely. Witmer's (1916) introduction of the possibility of congenital alexia existing to a very small degree in successful students is an important innovation that re-configures the diagnosis' potential operations: 'I run across college students, in their papers who must have a little congenital alexia' (Witmer, 1916: 190). This is a significant shift from Hinshelwood (1896: 1508, 1904) who had argued that it was only appropriate to apply the diagnosis in the most severe cases. While other researchers (and later Hinshelwood, 1907: 1232) began to advocate the possibility of milder cases, these were cases where the subject was still encountering educational problems, severe enough for them to be sent to see a medical specialist. The subjects that Witmer refers to do not seem to have encountered severe educational problems as they had been able to make it through the educational system and began attending college before the diagnosis of congenital aphasia was attached to their bodies. Witmer then outlines further details of students who encountered reading difficulties at college:

> For instance, there is a part of the brain which you may have studied, the medulla oblongata, and I have had students taking this course write down 'meddling obligato'. I have also found students who after taking a year of psychology, maybe two, don't know how to spell psychology, at least not in combinations like 'physiological psychology.' They just fall down in a heap like that boy when he tried to spell *girl*. (1916: 190)

Witmer compares the difficulties his students have in spelling frequently-used aspects of their technical vocabulary with the difficulties of the girl he discussed earlier in his paper as indicators of the way the diagnosis is conceptualised for him. The proposed teaching methods that Witmer advocates are very similar to those of the British ophthalmologists (Hinshelwood, 1902, 1912). He shuns the possibility of teaching a child accredited with congenital amnesia visualis verbalis by the 'word method' and advocates a method based upon the utilisation of sound, advocating the utilisation of intellectual attributes that are not understood as being defective to overcome reading difficulties—a method previously advocated by Hinshelwood (1902, 1912):

> My recommendation is that this boy be placed in a special class. He ought to be taken very well in hand. For example, I do think that in

the educational backwardness of this boy, one factor is faulty educational method. You can't teach a child who has any sort of defective memory cases by the word method. You might just as well give it up. In my opinion, all of these cases have to be taught by the A, B, C method,—beat into their heads. Give the man a good deal of sound analysis. Start him anew, and quit trying to teach him by the word method. For children who are somewhat deficient, I find that the word method throws them in confusion for several years. I think this boy can be taught some reading and writing. (1916: 191)

The recommendation that the boy should be placed in a special class departs from the strong criticism from the ophthalmologists concerning this method, who had insisted that children accredited with congenital reading difficulties should be taught alone, and apart from the mainstream class and the special class (Hinshelwood, 1912). When considered in conjunction with Witmer's (1916) framing of these characteristics as an unproblematic difference, the reach of separatist educational techniques is being extended as the techniques become deployed to smaller deviations from the norm. The criticisms of the word method mirror similar critical remarks made in earlier papers by the ophthalmologists.

The A, B, C method is advocated; similarly to Hinshelwood, an emphasis is again being placed upon diction, as this attribute is not hampered by the characteristics that amnesia visualis verbalis describes, to overcome the specific difficulty with reading. Witmer is hopeful that the boy can be taught some reading and writing; however, he is doubtful of a significant improvement being achieved:

> I don't think that this boy we have seen today will ever get over his defect, but he can get over it enough to get out of the feebleminded class, I don't know. He ought to be tried as though he was a normal child and were somewhat difficult to teach. He has got to be taken in hand exactly as we would take in hand a person who is said to have no ear for music. Such a boy can be trained to sing so other people could stand hearing him sing, but he couldn't earn much of a living by it. I think this boy could be trained that much in school subjects, and it looks as if he should be trained in a trade. (1916: 191)

This doubt is a change in tone from the ophthalmologists, who were keen to assert how a drastic improvement could be achieved (Hinshelwood

1900a; Nettleship, 1901). To Witmer it appeared unlikely that the subject would improve enough to leave the feeble-minded class. This difference in expectation shows that amenisa visualis verbalis performs a slightly different operation from congenital word-blindness, and perhaps accounts for Witmer's willingness to refer to the child as backward (Town, 1911: 177; Witmer, 1916: 184). In Chapter 5 I detailed expert after expert recommending that children accredited with a congenital reading difficulty were educated separately, in isolation and certainly not in the same class as the feeble-minded. Witmer still attempted to distinguish between those accredited as feebleminded, backward or defective, and those accredited with congenital aphasia, as he suggests that children accredited with congenital aphasia should be educated as if they were a normal child that was somewhat difficult to teach. Congenital reading difficulties are here constituted as a small variance from the norm. The possibility of small variances from an ever-growing number of norms facilitates technologies of power performing increasingly minute and specialist operations. Witmer suggests that the boy should be encouraged to learn a trade, where reading and writing will be less problematic. The full breadth of jobs would not be open to the boy and, for Witmer, it would be a mistake to educate him as such. There seems to be a contradiction here. At a clinical level Witmer considers children accredited with specific reading difficulties to be quite distinct from the feeble-minded, but when it comes to intravenous pedagogic practices he proposes to treat them in a similar way. It is unclear whether his doubt concerning the possibility of significant improvement is specific to this case or is a broader factor he associates with this diagnosis. While Witmer suggests that children accredited with specific reading difficulties can improve their reading, the prognosis of the writers associated with *The Psychological Clinic* is more pessimistic than the British ophthalmological writers. Additionally, Witmer has a more pessimistic view of the career options of those diagnosed with amnesia visualis verbalis to the British ophthalmologists' views of future job prospects for those diagnosed with congenital word-blindness.

Beyond *The Psychological Clinic*

In 1921 Fildes published 'A Psychological Inquiry Into the Nature of the Condition Known as Congenital Word-blindness' in the journal *Brain*. This article furthered the repositioning of specific congenital reading difficulties as a psychological problem. Unlike the previous psychological papers (Town, 1911; Witmer 1907a, 1907b, 1916) discussed earlier in this chapter the terminological device, congenital word-blindness, is deployed here despite reservations about its utilisation:

> The aim of the investigation about to be described was to discover something of the psychological characteristics of the condition commonly called by the misleading term of congenital word-blindness—a condition which shows itself most clearly in the subjects' extreme difficulty, or even total failure, in learning to read, and appears to be closely related to the various forms of acquired alexia met with commonly as the result of brain injury in later life. (1921: 286)

Like so many writers before him Fildes finds fault with the term 'congenital-word-blindness'. For Fildes, however, it is the emphasis on the *congenital* element of the term, and not the blindness, which was misleading. The adjective, *congenital*, downplays the influence of environmental factors, such as education, which can improve a subject's reading ability. Fildes's suggestion that there is a closeness between the acquired and congenital forms of word-blindness contrasts with the strong attempts to distinguish between the two that previously-discussed ophthalmologists had made (Hinshelwood, 1896, 1900a, 1902, 1907; Thomas, 1905). This is similar to the move made by Witmer (1907b).

Fildes provided a description of the variety of intelligence tests that he deployed to make the diagnosis: '(a) with the Stanford revision of the Binet scale, in order to get some idea of their general mental capacity, and (b) with various recognized reading tests, in order to get an estimate of their reading power' (1921: 286–7) through which a visible diagram of the subject's intelligence could be drawn. The combination of these tests, utilised in assemblage with general reading tests, allowed for the construction of visible, and, more importantly, measurable profiles, of the subject's reading difficulties to be outlined. Fildes describes the advantages of being able to deploy tests that measured an individual's ability with reading specifically, rather than having to depend upon a general intelligence test:

> Testing for reading power in particular revealed also a great variation in the ability of the subjects. Some of them could recognize no single letter, word or figure with any certainty; others could read simple words and knew all letters and figures well. It was estimated, however, that no child was less than four years retarded in reading ability

and some of them showed retardation much greater than this. Even the children who could read best had a marked difficulty in writing from memory words which they could read—they could not spell. (1921: 287)

Fildes records that the results of the intelligence tests of individuals diagnosed as congenitally word-blind did not reflect the degree of their difficulty with the lexicon: '[n]o relationship existed between the subjects' intelligence quotients and their power in reading. Two of the worst readers were the least intelligent and most intelligent boys' (1921: 287). Fildes clearly indicates that individuals could be vastly intelligent while still having incredible difficulties with specific educational attributes, such as reading or spelling. Their difficulties could also be very particular within these attributes. For instance, he details how there were particular words they would often confuse with others. Crucially, a specifically pronounced difficulty with reading does not necessarily result, for Fildes, in heightened intelligence. The eleven experiments conducted by Fildes attempted to analyse three potential psychological theories of congenital word-blindness:

(1) A theory which assumes the existence of definitely localized and circumscribed visual and auditory word-centres in the brain, the destruction or isolation of which will destroy language in either its visual or its auditory aspect;

(2) A theory which interprets word-blindness as only one symptom in a general lowering of mental ability; and

(3) One which attributes the condition to a more specialized lowering of power in the primary visual centres, rendering true visual perception of words and of other complex sense-data difficult. (1921: 286)

Kussmaul's (1877) proposition that two hemispheres of the brain serve different cognitive functions is essentially re-articulated by Fildes affirming the 'existence of definitely localized and circumscribed visual and auditory word-centres in the brain' (Fildes, 1921: 286). The experiments conducted by Fildes were therefore attempting to establish what the cerebral difference that causes specific reading difficulties are. The aetiology proposed here is somewhere between that of the British ophthalmologists and the researchers associated with *The Psychological*

Clinic. Fildes's experimental psychological approach identified the possibility of congenital reading difficulties as being engendered by an alternative way of processing information. The diagrams drawn by these experiments opened the possibility of describing, assessing and managing variance in the way in which humans process information:

> the experiments indicate that the cause of the failure to associate, as well as to retain, sounds and forms, lies to some degree in this primary disability of the auditory or visual regions, resulting as it does in the failure of the forms or sounds presented to gain any meaning. (Fildes, 1921: 307)

Fildes suggests that differing levels of development in different regions of the brain generate a congenital reading difficulty (this is similar to the aetiologies put forward by Kussmaul (1877), Hinshewlood (1895) and Witmer (1907b)). For Fildes (1921), an individual who is accredited with congenital reading difficulties as a 'primary disability' will be resultant of the difficulty in establishing a connection between written symbols and auditory information. This therefore leads to a difficulty in developing the skills needed to read. For Fildes (1921), 'congenital' or 'developmental' reading disabilities result from the difference in the development between different regions in the brain. This a distinct diagnostic category to the others proposed thus far. The thesis presented by Fildes (1921) was very similar to the one presented by Samuel Orton (1925). The main focus of Orton's text is to produce a diagram of the dyslexic brain as distinct from the normal brain. Orton is interested in neurological differentiation between the 'dyslexic brain' and the 'normal brain'.

Blanchie Minogue's 1927 article illustrates how children who were thought to have difficulties with reading now began to be referred to educational practitioners and psychologists, rather than ophthalmologists, suggesting that the link between psychologists and educationalists had now been firmly established: 'Recently there was brought to the child guidance clinic at Nyack, a girl of twelve years, with the complaint that she failed to get along in school. The case was referred by the school principal who felt convinced that the girl was a mental defective' (Minogue, 1927: 226). The jurisdiction over word-blindness had shifted from the medical–ophthalmological axis to the two-pronged psychological–educational axis. The evidence I have drawn from the literature suggests that the psychologists were more readily able to articulate educational apparatus into their programmes, practices and procedures. Minogue's description of his patient illustrates an increased emphasis upon hereditary factors not found in Thomas (1905), Rutherford (1909) or Town (1911).

> A. B. was born in New England, June 23, 1914. The family history was negative for nervous and mental diseases. The parents were obviously of good intelligence and the two older children, one in high school two and a half years, and the other in junior high school at eleven years, appeared superior. The patient herself presented a history typical of that usually found in mental defectives. She could not make progress in school and was wholly unable to read. She had been advanced in spite of this until, at twelve years, she was in the fifth grade. Here, as in the preceding grades, she did excellent work in arithmetic, but nothing in reading and spelling. Geography, history and language, being so dependent on reading, were likewise poor. In personality the child was rather excitable and very sensitive. She preferred to play with younger and smaller children. The physical examination was negative. She was a well developed girl, and very attractive. There was no history of injury or infectious illnesses. (1927: 226)

The emphasis on the subject being very attractive is noteworthy and perhaps adds to her status as being 'deserving' of the specific guidance and training she was to receive. In addition to this, the description of the family history that presents the family as being intelligent, with her two older siblings being referred to as 'superior', develops this trope further still. This emphasis suggests that she was considered to be a useful resource that could be cultivated. Her ability to advance through school even though she could not read implies that she was deserving, as she was evidently intellectually advanced, being able to use her other intellectual attributes to substitute for the areas where she had difficulties. Minogue notes that the principal of the school was then contacted with advice on how to continue with the girl's education, illustrating that connections between psychology and educationalists had now been well established:

> The principal of the school was notified and an attempt is being made to secure special teaching for the girl. The recommendations in her case are:
>
> 1. That the child, who is now right-handed, be taught to use her left hand as a means of developing the corresponding center on

the other side of the brain. This method is advocated by both Dr. Orton 1 of Iowa City and Dr. McCready of Pittsburg.

2. That special instruction in reading and spelling be given. Painstaking drilling in the fundamentals, always with the realization that the patient can read letters and that she learns best through auditory channels, should produce good results.

3. That the child be encouraged in every possible way. She has suffered so long and so keenly from her disability that she is much disturbed emotionally. Wise and sympathetic handling should do much to improve her stability.

The prognosis in this case appears unusually good. The child has a decided advantage in her good environment and fine intelligence level. Added to this is the fact that she understands her own condition and is gamely determined to overcome it. It is regrettable that this case is so recent that nothing has as yet been accomplished in the teaching project. It is suggestive, of course, of the number of other children, backward in school, and presenting somewhat the picture of a mental defective, who may be retarded on this account. It is probable that word-blindness occurs frequently among the feeble-minded, but in such cases a diagnosis, although interesting, is not so vital as in the instance of a bright child. Even if this disability occurs in but one of every two thousand normal children, as is estimated, it seems reasonable that cases should appear from time to time at our clinics. (1927: 229–30)

Minogue's description continues the operation (Hinshelwood, 1896, 1900a, 1902; Witmer, 1907b, 1916) of establishing a difference between children accredited as feeble-minded, backward or defective, and those diagnosed with congenital word-blindness. Interventions into the child's education and, indeed, her general conduct are recommended. Recommendations such as teaching her to use her left hand were considered as a technique for intervening directly upon her brain, fostering the development of the corresponding cortex. This follows recommendations already developed by McCready (1925) and Orton (1925). Technologies can thus be deployed upon the flesh of the body with the intent of producing effects upon the workings of the brain.

The educational programme advocated is described as 'painstaking'; we can assume that this is not only for the child in question, but also for those concerned with educating her. This painstaking programme will be concerned with 'the fundamentals'—most likely to be language and maths. It has been established that the girl in question learns best through auditory channels—suggesting that instructors need to find the most productive method for teaching the particular child in question. At this point the diagnosis of congenital word-blindness appears to be continuing to facilitate the microscopic approach to the production of bodies, where individual intellectual attributes are targeted by educational apparatus, in a specific and precise way. This is, perhaps, a further development from a bio-politics of the population (Foucault, 1979) to a microscopically focused bio-politics where individual attributes are managed at an atomic level to facilitate the bio-political cultivation of the population. This necessitates the segmentation of the population into increasingly specific categories with characteristics that can be cultivated and managed, allowing the specific goals of a rationality of government to be achieved.

Charles Ford's article in *The Psychological Clinic*, 'A Case of Congenital Word-Blindness Showing its Social Implications', is the first of three articles published in 1928 in this journal, evidencing that within the sub-discipline of clinical psychology congenital reading difficulties were now a fully accepted area of study. The article is also noteworthy as it documents a terminological shift, with the earlier terminological devices deployed by Witmer (1907a, 1907b, 1916) and Town (1911) dropped in favour of a return to the category of congenital word-blindness. Ford follows the path already laid by Witmer (1907a, 1907b) in emphasising the relation between aphasia and congenital word-blindness, which, for a time, had been less prominent in the literature:

> The matter of congenital word blindness has been recognized since Dr. Morgan first reported a case in 1896 and so named it because of its similarity to aphasic word blindness. Since this time many cases of reading disorders have been reported, some of which are included in the bibliography appended. Three main factors appear to be common to the congenitally word blind. (1) They cannot read words although they can read other symbols as music and letters; (2) they have no other outstanding mental or physical defect and (3) they can be taught to read the if correct method is found. (1928: 73)

The institution of a relation between a previously related diagnosis aphasic word blindness (which had become less emphasised in the ophthalmological literature) acted to strengthen the jurisdiction that psychology was developing over congenital word-blindness. This was a move that had already been made by Witmer (1907b, 1916) and Town (1911) in the very same journal. Like Hinshelwood, Ford (1928) states that no other physical or mental defect can be present for a case of word-blindness to be confidently diagnosed. The diagnosis is once again concerned with describing an isolated and specific difficulty—even more crucially, a difficulty that can be overcome.

Ford has thus added to the clinical criteria that the patient can overcome word-blindness as one of the criteria for the patient being diagnosed as congenitally word-blind. Being a malleable, improvable subject is one of the criteria for being distinguished from those accredited as feeble-minded, backward or defective by acquiring the diagnosis of congenital word-blindness. Word-blindness is here modulated into a technology to differentiate between valuable capital and worthless capital.

> The condition is rare and yet Wallin reports that the found 4.1 per cent who could be so diagnosed out of 2,774 children examined who were not making satisfactory school progress. This is the highest estimate of its incidence we have found in the literature, but any who are familiar with school clinic examinations know that reading defects account for a sizeable number of retardates. (Ford, 1928: 73)

It is intriguing that Ford presents the characteristics here as rare, as it is this rarity that has hitherto been called into question by so many writers already discussed (Hinshelwood, 1896, 1900a, 1904; Nettleship, 1901). Estimates of the number of children who could be accredited with this condition reach a high point in the literature discussed, as congenital word-blindness becomes seen as an increasingly common condition amongst school children. Ford seems to be suggesting that large numbers of children could be diagnosed with congenital word-blindness, but that this diagnosis should be reserved for specific circumstances. This is similar to the introduction by Hinshelwood (1907: 1232) of pure congenital word-blindness to maintain the potency of the diagnosis' operation:

> Despite the fact the condition is well known and found rather regularly in school clinics the school, implications have not been the subject matter of any the articles. Three main ideas are involved in presenting the following case. The first is to present a case study showing definitely the conditions surrounding the case both as a matter of history and measured results. The second is to give a technique in the examinations of the congenital word blind. The third is to show that the described condition is a cause of severe school and social maladjustment. (1928: 73)

While reams have now been written on congenital word-blindness, no texts, according to Ford, have been published identifying the social implications of the characteristics the diagnosis encompasses. Ford proposes that children who have the characteristics of congenital word-blindness, but did not receive a diagnosis early enough, may experience social difficulties at school. A case study is then presented, which details how a particular boy came under Ford's auspices. This boy was brought to the attention of psychological experts owing to the recommendation by a juvenile court, which detailed the boy's problematic behaviour and his social difficulties:

> Paul was referred to the Bureau by one of the large juvenile courts of the state because he was guilty of lying, stealing from home and school, truancy and being a disturber in school. Test such as these were not new to Paul as he had previously been given psychological examinations in May, 1922, and again in February 1927. (1928: 74)

The negative character assessment, and his history with the juvenile courts, is now juxtaposed with Ford's experiences of the child, which are quite different. Ford appears to be concerned with suggesting that the boy's difficulties are social and that if he is treated properly he is a perfectly well-behaved boy:

> Paul is a loveable boy, attractive in appearance, orderly in his habits, and at least during his stay with us, he has been thoroughly trustworthy. He is not overly phlegmatic and yet he is unique and reticent. The whole impression of the lad rather leads one to feel that he is a lad of satisfactory intelligence equipment who has been made to feel inferior and is therefore rather afraid to let go. We have no evidence of his fighting, quarrelling, masturbating nor bed wetting while here. (1928: 76)

Paul's physical condition and character are described in detail. IQ tests at various ages are given. Like Minogue (1927), as discussed earlier, Paul's good looks are affirmed, again marking him as deserving—a body worthy of further attention, of cultivation. The second examination contained a note: 'Marked disability to read; cannot read even first grade work. Recognizes only short words. Should have careful examination of the eyes' (Ford, 1928: 77–8). Ophthalmological examinations are being posited as a necessary technology in the process of identifying the aetiology of the particular reading disability in question, to exclude the possibility of the origin of the localised difficulty with reading, being ocular in it's character. Ophthalmology is then articulated by Ford as part of the machinery that psychology utilised to diagnose bodies as congenitally word-blind. The position of ophthalmology in the machinery of government concerned with diagnosing bodies with congenital word-blindness had shifted. Ford then gives further details to the social implications for the diagnosis he had begun to elaborate earlier:

> His behaviour problems have apparently increased with each succeeding year in school. In kindergarten, so far as can be learned, his problems were nil. As soon as he entered the grades he became an even greater problem. As a teacher indicated in a letter previously quoted, no teacher he has had has been able to fathom his difficulty. During his enrolment at _____ Park School, he started truancy, but so far as we can learn, this was not until his second year in the first grade. (1928: 81)

This boy's difficulties are elaborated on later in the paper:

> When transferred to X Road school his problems continued to increase. Stealing was added to his list as was gross lying. True, there was a different environment in his new home but this was made worse because he couldn't read. He tells us that his uncle, who is 14 years old, calls him 'dummy' because he doesn't read, and he also says his playmates 'kid' him about his difficulty. (1928: 81–2)

We are informed that with each preceding year of school, Paul's behaviour has worsened. As the work had become more difficult for Paul he had responded by acting in a poorer fashion. If bad behaviour is associated with children accredited with congenital word-blindness, then an additional reason for improving these children's difficulties with reading is apparent in order to allow for the education of the rest of the class to continue unabated without disruptive conduct. Further evidence is provided to the argument that children accredited with congenital word-blindness are unfairly treated (Hinshelwood, 1896), suffering insults and other negative attacks, which, as documented in this case, seem to have had an adverse affect on Paul's behaviour. The report documents how his behaviour worsened as he progressed through school, alluding to the possibility that this had augmented as he felt increasingly alienated from his schooling.

Ford continues to paint an extremely sympathetic picture of Paul, suggesting that the misunderstanding of educational characteristics and the subsequent way he was treated accounted for his bad behaviour:

'His teachers apparently are out of sympathy with him, his father and stepmother think he is deficient mentally, his grandmother is weary of caring for him. Small wonder then that Paul is maladjusted' (1928: 82). His family's perceptions of him and the resultant treatment were now put forward as an explanation for Paul's maladjustment and bad behaviour. The implication is put forward by Ford that fairer treatment would have been a way of avoiding the behavioural problems that Paul exhibited during his schooling.

> There is no known organic defect. Visual sensitivity and hearing are normal. The English language has always been spoken in his home. His parents and grandparents read for pleasure. (1928: 83)

Ford details that he is suffering from no linguistic disadvantage and that he comes from a literate household, where reading is engaged in as an activity for pleasure, and that he is physically able to read. All other possible aetiologies are therefore excluded, apart from a congenital reading difficulty. Intelligence tests are here deployed to identify the specific character of his difficulty, and are subsequently utilised as evidence of the boy's otherwise intelligent character:

> Whether or not his intelligence is normal is a question if test results alone are considered. However, he has evidenced such thoroughly normal behaviour while with us that we feel sure his level is at least as high or higher than test results would indicate. Test level, however, is sufficiently high to indicate he has enough intelligence to read. Throughout the entire period of examining he was on the defensive. He was used to being considered dual and this has undoubtedly influenced his score as it surely did his behaviour. (1928: 83)

The case being presented here suggests that because the boy was considered in a negative manner he learnt to act in such a way, responding in his behaviour to the way people conceived of him. Ford considers that his alienation from his environment permeated his body and his behaviour responded to the negative perceptions that people had of him. This leads Ford to suggest that congenital word-blindness or congenital dyslexia should have been seen as a social maladjustment; this is a unique position amongst the writers I have so far discussed:

> We cannot help but feel more emphasis should be placed on the matter of congenital word-blindness and congenital dyslexia as an element

in social maladjustment. Here is another clear case of, at least average home conditions, an approximately normal boy in level and function, where school and social maladjustment is the result of the condition. He has lost the sympathy and understanding of the home and school. He had been made to feel inferior by being held back in school and chided by his associates and his recourse is fighting, stealing, truancy, etc. None of these manifestations have been gross but they are irritating and serve only to make him appear even worse than he is. (1928: 83)

The description implies that the boy's internalisation of the perception of inferiority, propagated by his school and his family, have led to increasingly anti-social behaviour—we are told that he has simply become resigned to the environment he has been placed in. Positioning social maladjustment as a possible aetiology for congenital word-blindness departs from every other aetiology reviewed thus far as they all rely upon the assumption that a particular region of the brain is defective. This provides an illustration of how a diagram of the human, seen through the eyes technical instruments, is making visible particular human characteristics as impairment categories.

Ford (1928) goes on to elaborate how this social maladjustment can be overcome. We learn that Paul's body responded to positive cultivation and management, his behaviour improved and he indicated an interest in learning:

That these statements of feelings of inferiority and its compensation are not pure hypothesis is shown by the fact that Paul was maladjusted at home where he was considered dull and he gets along well here where he is not considered dull. The lad is not inferior to the bulk of boys now about him. He is made to feel capable and he responds by being faithful to many trusts. He has caused no trouble in a group who are here because of troublesomeness, and who are trouble makers here. He has been in no fights; he has not lied and last of all he is keenly interested and alive to things about him. (1928: 83–4)

Paul has been reconstituted as a body that is amenable to the effects of educational technologies. Intervening to improve the reading abilities of children accredited as having a congenital reading difficulty is shown to have also improved his behaviour. Ford highlights how successful educationalists have been in teaching those diagnosed as congenitally word-blind to read:

One of the most hopeful elements in the matter of congenital word-blindness is that all reported cases have been taught to read. Reasoning by analogy we hope then Paul's problems can be minimized, because he too can be taught to read if the proper method can be found and the proper encouragement maintained. (1928: 84)

Bodies accredited as congenitally word-blind have been marked as deserving of attention, specialised and often given separate attention because they can, despite their specific difficulty, become productive (Ford, 1928; Nettleship, 1901). Ford notes that all the reported cases have been taught to read. Bodies hitherto seen as without economic potential were transformed into a cultivable resource. The rationale of government now appears to be 'we must not only learn how to maximise the power of the population, but how to transform bodies that have hitherto been seen as without economic potential into useable capital'.

Conclusion

The psychologists who researched reading difficulties produced a diagnostic category that was extremely similar to congenital word-blindness. While Ford (1928) showed an awareness of Hinshelwood and the other British ophthalmologists' research on these topics, Witmer (1907a, 1907b, 1916), who established *The Psychological Clinic* journal, seems to be unaware of this earlier work. A variety of different terminologies were used to describe their category: 'visual deafness' 'amnesia visualis verbalis' and, finally, 'congenital word-blindness'. The differences in articulation of the diagnosis are partially concerned with disciplinary conventions, with the psychologists being in a better position to utilise a wide variety of technologies from other disciplines in assemblage to make their version of the diagnosis the most veritable. These circumstances resulted in the relations with other congenital aphasias being re-emphasised. The crucial difference between the writers associated with *The Psychological Clinic* and the ophthalmologists, who were the focus of my earlier chapters, is the greater emphasis within *The Psychological Clinic* on establishing relations with schools and other educational institutions. The psychologists associated with *The Psychological Clinic* were more successful than the ophthalmologists and were able to disperse their conception of the diagnosis across a wider range of educational institutions and schools. Through being able to operate in assemblage with a greater number of technologies of power, the writers associated with *The Psychological Clinic*, were able to fashion their version of the diagnosis as part of a more effective machinery of government.

While, on the one hand, describing more exact and seemingly less problematic difficulties with reading, and comparing these characteristics with left-handedness, Witmer, on the other hand, indicates that some pupils would not be able to leave the special room, while others may go on to college. This illustrates that the diagnosis simultaneously becomes concerned with rehabilitating individuals whose difficulties are moderate enough for them to go to college, while also endorsing educational segregation for those children whose difficulties are pronounced enough to become apparent during their schooling. In Witmer's view, some of these children's difficulties are so pronounced that they will not be able to leave the special room. The bio-politics of Witmer and the other writers associated with *The Psychological Clinic* are distinct from that of the British ophthalmologists, taking a more negative view of the population that their diagnosis described, while concurrently wishing to help those with less pronounced characteristics overcome their difficulties by utilising the same methods that had been advocated by Hinshelwood and his associates. These differences in the bio-political operation of the diagnosis should be related to the differing character of the eugenic movements in the USA and the UK, which resulted in these categories being formed in dialogue with strategies of government that conceived of the body of the individual and the body of the population in distinct ways. The psychological machinery described in this chapter was gaining significant social and political influence. By working in assemblage with this machinery the diagnosis was able perform a more subtle operation on the complexly diagrammed body that was emerging. In the next chapter I shall describe how congenital reading difficulties became a concern of educationalists, illustrating how a machinery of government concerned with managing educational difference was formed.

7
The Problem of Producing Literate Subjects: Education and Specific Reading Difficulties

This chapter describes the work of a variety of authors whose writings on reading in educational journals made the school an increasingly hospitable site for a diagnosis such as congenital word-blindness to be deployed. The processes by which children learnt to read; the importance of these bodies acquiring the ability to read in order to develop a more advanced understanding of various subjects; the development of a concern that some pupils had a pronounced difficulty with reading; techniques for improving overall reading rates of a class and individuals accredited as having a difficulty; tests used to examine reading ability; the perceived social–cultural benefits of reading; and the emergence of specific techniques for educating children accredited with congenital word-blindness are all discussed in the journals from which I have drawn the following discussion.

The purpose of these discussions is to provide a broader context of the discursive and non-discursive formations that were forming around the practice of reading at the turn the twentieth century. This context will complement the analysis presented in the preceding chapters regarding the formation of particular strategies of government and the importance that I have suggested a literate population had for the goals of some these strategies. The paramount position of reading in education is established, and further evidence is gathered to support the contention that literate bodies were becoming ever more necessary to emerging machineries of government as the twentieth century progressed, as our communicative capacities were increasingly articulated into production. Particular attention is paid to the writings of Clara Schmitt, as she published the first article on congenital word-blindness in a teaching journal (1914). This article is also the first time a considered and detailed approach to the education of those accredited as having a congenital reading difficulty appeared in academic journal. This approach was concerned with improving the literacy of those diagnosed with congenital word-blindness. Her article on the testing of mental ability is thus analysed in some depth, as it is of particular relevance to understanding how the machinery of education became hospitable to specific reading difficulties. The majority of the other articles discussed have been culled from the *Elementary School Journal*, where Schmitt published the aforementioned paper. In what follows I try and describe how a concern with reading developed within this journal and educational practice in general, as well as how reading difficulties became a concern for these professionals. I will therefore illustrate how it became possible to speak of congenital word-blindness within a particular professional grouping. The preceding chapters have been concerned with the conditions of formation for congenital reading difficulties in the clinical disciplines of medicine, ophthalmology and psychology. The discussion now moves away from analysing a technology of governments' conditions of formation to a study of the process of its veridiction, describing how congenital word-blindness became a deployable technology in the pursuit of cultivating a literate population. This chapter describes how a strategy of proliferating the skill of reading onto bodies that initially found reading hard to develop was facilitated by educationalists taking up the technologies of government that were fashioned by psychologists.

The Veneration of Reading and its Importance to Education

In educational literature reading is venerated, as its centrality to most methods of instruction necessitates reverence from educational practitioners. Bowden (1911) discusses how reading had become second nature for many adults. For Bowden, reading had become comparable to walking—something that we do out of instinct. Adults forget the process that they went through to become equipped with the ability to read and the complex character of this process. Bowden therefore wishes to remind his readers of the difficulty they had in acquiring the ability to read printed symbols:

> The adult gives no more thought to his reading than he gives to his walking. The process has become automatic; when he sees the printed symbols he reads in spite of himself. He can no more tell how he reads than he can tell how he walks; he simply reads. He has so far

forgotten the time and energy he spent mastering the process that he is not even aware of its complexity. (1911: 21)

Bowden argues that adults have forgotten the complexity of the muscular process involved in reading. This is why the index finger of a beginner reader often traces an imaginary line under the text as they read. At first the body finds it hard to learn to read, fixating over each line. However, it is necessary to train the body to be able to stay fixed on the line in question. Learning to read can be a tiring and laborious process, as it is a refined and technical process:

> Reading sometimes tires his brain and sometimes tires his eyes; further in the analysis he does not go. He may think that his eyes do not move across the page with each line but that he takes in two or more lines at once; he may believe that the movement is a continuous one and that he experiences no difficulty in gauging the length of the line or in fixating any given point in the line. When the psychologist tells him that he reads but a line at a time, that the movement across the page is a succession of short movements and brief pauses, and that even after the movements have become automatic, the eyes sometimes fail to fixate the correct point, he realizes that learning to read is a difficult task for the eyes, and he understands why the beginner's finger follows the line word by word as he reads. (1911: 21)

As reading is a complex multi-movement process of considerable difficulty, it is almost expected that some individuals will encounter problems trying to develop this skill. For Bowden, the fact some people find it difficult to learn to read is not surprising. Educationalists, though, have to be reminded that reading is a skill that is time-consuming and difficult to acquire, engendering sympathy in them for those children who find it difficult to acquire this skill. This is necessary, as educationalists have often forgotten the laborious process that they, too, had to partake in.

William Gray (whose work on testing reading abilities is given a more detailed treatment below) describes reading as being one of the most important factors in determining promotions through the lower grades of American schooling, as it becomes increasingly central in accessing the broader curriculum (1919: 336). The central importance of reading to schooling is affirmed, as it is necessary to learn to read to be able to receive instruction later in school as the education system becomes increasingly reliant upon the independent study of books to facilitate the development of specialised knowledge. Reading is an attribute that must be proliferated throughout the population of a school, to facilitate the future deployment of a variety of technologies of government that require the subject to be literate:

> Reading was selected as the basis for this study because of its large importance in the elementary-school curriculum. In the lower grades ability to read is commonly adopted as the most important factor in determining promotions. In the upper grades ability to study content subjects intelligently is prerequisite to rapid progress. An investigation of reading assumes increased importance when the relation of reading ability to the various phases of school work is fully recognized. (Gray, 1919: 336)

The research Gray conducted identified what social and educational attributes teachers believed the instruction of reading developed in their pupils. Gray asked teachers what was the most desirable qualities that the instruction of reading developed among their pupils. A variety of desirable qualities and useful habits were facilitated by learning how to read:

1. Ability to get thought from a printed page.
2. Speed in reading.
3. Formation of dictionary habit.
4. Increased vocabulary.
5. Interest in current news.
6. Formation of library habit.
7. Creation of standards of taste.
8. Appreciation of notable pieces of literature.
9. Interest in subject read.

(1919: 345)

Cultivating the ability to read allows for an individual to acquire information and skills independently from an instructor. Interest in literature and the news is fostered, and vocabulary is expanded. Through learning to read, the body was made amenable to a variety of information, and an interest in current affairs, literature and library habit were thought to be developed. Making a body literate expands the number of capillaries of government that could be applied to the body. Gray then asked the teachers how the work they did in their grade contributed to the aforementioned results. Their replies show the reliance upon so many aspects of the educational machinery, on the ability to read printed text. The positive effects of reading on a pupil's habits and character meant that, for Gray, reading was an essential way of proliferating positive characteristics, interests and morals throughout the population. A philanthropic view of spreading literacy throughout the population seems to be held by the teachers Gray interviewed:

1. Systematic training in silent reading develops the ability to master thought.
2. This, too, when made a competitive class exercise, increases the speed of reading.
3. The use of the dictionary is encouraged in the preparation of reading lessons and also in the silent-reading class exercise when speed is not an objective.
4. Fitting the right meanings of words to their uses in sentences increases a pupil's vocabulary. Extensive use of these words is encouraged in spoken and written composition.
5. The interest of the class is aroused in matters of general interest, such as gardening, food economy, the Liberty Loan, or Red Cross work, to such an extent that clippings from daily papers are brought and read, or passed about, or posted on the bulletin board.
6. During a part of the term the class has met once a week in the library and the pupils have taken out and returned the books which they have selected to read. These are recommended by one to another, and sometimes a report is given by one pupil to the other members of the class.
7. The encouragement of a better class of fiction really does implant in the child a feeling for better books.
8. Some selections are read merely for appreciation, sometimes by the teacher in morning exercises, sometimes recited by a pupil, or again memorized by a class.
9. The interest aroused by reading such a book as Burroughs' Birds and Bees is of great importance, and the influence of extensive reading of this type is far-reaching. A boy wants to explain how he made his canoe, a girl produces a birch-bark booklet from Vermont, and so the experiences multiply. This interest may take the form of a problem or question. A class discussion ensues, or an extended investigation follows.

(1919: 344–5)

Reading, for Guilfoile (1921), much like the teachers who responded to Gray's aforementioned question, had many benefits that went beyond simply the transmission of information. Moreover, reading is the primary device through which an individual's imagination can be developed, and it is essential to the development of independent thought and reflection. Being equipped with the ability to read encourages the development of autonomous working and fosters an interest in a variety of subjects. Facilitating the development of aesthetic values, such as the ability to discern between a good book and a bad one, the learning of these literary values and mastering how to use the public library are also revered. The importance that Guilfoile accords to these values that can be acquired by developing the right relationship with texts underlies why acquiring a high level of reading comprehension was necessary if a body was going to have to be imbued with a high degree of cultural capital and social standing:

> aside from the gain in reading ability, the class gained other things of at least equal value. They learned the use of the public library and the care of books that are public property. They learned to some extent literary values. They can distinguish a good book from a poor one. They have become acquainted with a volume of literary material with which they should have come in contact in their earlier childhood, both through their own reading and through listening to others. They have found for themselves new worlds which they can explore independently. (1921: 131)

For the writers discussed here, reading is the most technically effective pedagogical device, but also provides an additional bio-political procedure imbuing those who undertake it with numerous desirable social traits: once literacy has been kneaded into a body, the flesh becomes increasingly malleable. Guilfoile seems quite intoxicated by the benefits of reading, finding the development of this skill in students as necessary. This is not just because she is concerned with producing the most economically productive students. Rather, she chooses to focus on giving students the chance to encounter the many gifts that literature has to offer.

The Measurement of Reading

Intelligence tests allowed for the cognitive abilities of individuals and populations to be mapped, analysed and compared. Congenital word-blindness, and later dyslexia, relied heavily upon the ability to measure specific cognitive abilities, and illustrate a discrepancy between them.

Throughout the nineteenth century, in the wake of the invention of normality, the human body was subjected to an ever-growing array of techniques for measuring bodies (Davis, 1995; Ewald, 1990, 1991; Hacking, 1982, 1990). Tests were primarily devised to measure reading ability, although in some cases they were used to measure a variety of different attributes of reading. The standard test was one of these. The purpose and place of standard tests is outlined by Courtis (1914). They should be precise and simple, as it is their simplicity that made them great measurers of educational aptitude. Standard tests differ from examinations, as they are concerned with evaluating an individual's progress across a particular programme of study. Examinations are typically re-written with every session, and standard tests would remain the same every time they were deployed. Standard tests are not made to measure the success a pupil achieved in a particular curricula, but, instead, an attribute of education. These tests were technologies of power that facilitated the measurement of the aptitude of a pupil in relation to a particular skill. Working in assemblage with the norm, standard tests allowed for power to be generalized from the body of the individual to the body of the population (Ewald, 1990: 141). Furthermore, this allowed the body of the individual to be managed in such a fashion as to cultivate the body of the population. Courtis's description of the standard test supports this notion and describes how they differ from examinations:

> Standard tests in education are rulers for the measurement of educational products; tools for research work. They should be differentiated from the ordinary examinations on the one hand and the more rigid and formal measurements of the experimental psychologists on the other. An examination, for instance, is supposed to show whether or not the individual has successfully completed a prescribed course of work. Examinations are complex, are usually made afresh each time they are given, and only in the most general sense may the conditions under which they are given said to be controlled. (1914: 374)

The operation standard tests are able to perform upon both individual bodies and the body of the population is described by Courtis:

> In the writer's thinking, the functions of standard educational tests are four: (a) to secure information that will enable school authorities to formulate in objective terms the ends to be attained in any

educational process; (b) to measure the efficiency of methods designed to produce the desired results; (c) to determine the factors and laws which condition learning and teaching; (d) to furnish data that will enable comparisons of school with school, and teacher with teacher for purposes of supervisory control to be made upon scientific, impersonal, objective bases. (1914: 375)

Technologies that allow for reading abilities of individual students to be measured, to be modelled, facilitate comparisons between student's distinct characteristics. This allowed for students to be described as remedial, as standard tests were used to identify how far below the expected level a student fell. Standard tests also made it possible for a child to be described as remedial in one area, but not in another. Information of generalised results could also be provided to school authorities, allowing for the government of reading to become more systematic. Courtis describes how experimental studies have shown that educational difficulties are regularly the result of a difficulty with reading. Establishing tests for the specific purpose of studying the various aspects of the skills that are taught under the rubric English became imperative.

> Recent experimental studies have seemed to show that the chief difficulties are closely connected with the abilities involved in reading. It has become imperative, therefore, to determine standard rates of reading and of comprehension; but in giving tests for this purpose it was found that the material secured could be scored in so many other ways of value that the group of tests has been combined into a single series under the head of 'English Tests.' These have been issued on the same co-operative basis followed in the arithmetic work, and are now being standardized by teachers and superintendents in different parts of the country. (1914: 378)

Reading difficulties were found to be the most prevalent of educational difficulties, and the centrality of reading in schooling makes this particularly problematic. Reading difficulties are thus signalled as a priority for educational researchers to study. Judd elaborates the usefulness of standard tests, as described by Courtis, for evaluating whether schools are efficiently carrying out the task at hand. The measurement of reading ability allows for standards to be set that have to be achieved before progress to the next grade can be approved. Reading tests therefore facilitate the development of more complex machinery and strategies of governing the population of a school:

> With this definition of the meaning of standards in mind, let us con-sider some of the comparative problems which are of importance in the teaching of reading in the elementary school. In the first place, it is obvious that a comparison of different grades in the same school system is a matter of great importance. If the child shows adequate progress as he passes from the second to the third grade, from the third to the fourth grade, and so on, we may be satisfied that the school is doing efficient work even if the ability to read at any given point is in the absolute not great. Or, to put the matter in another way, the grade which is steadily improving shows a higher degree of efficiency than a grade which is improving less rapidly, even though the grade which is improving less rapidly shows a fair degree of abil-ity. In preparing our test, therefore, we should aim to determine the rate of improvement during the different grades. (Judd, 1914: 367)

Judd describes Courtis's argument, which states that rates of writing are an integral part of many reading examinations. In the many articles con-cerned with difficulties with reading, a concern with writing difficulties is only regularly found in the British articles concerned with congenital word-blindness. However, it is found less frequently in articles on reading difficulties in *The Elementary School Journal* and *The Psychological Clinic*:

> Mr. Courtis has shown in his tests the importance of the child's rate of writing as an element in any test which calls upon the child to reproduce ideas that he has acquired through reading. The child who writes slowly is disadvantaged in comparison with the child who writes rapidly, so that our definition of a child's ability to reproduce ideas should undoubtedly include ultimately his ability to write. The difficulty which is here encountered can be overcome so far as indi-vidual tests are concerned by allowing children to reproduce orally the ideas acquired. The teacher has now to note those ideas which are correctly reproduced and those which are omitted. Part of the difficulty can also be eliminated by giving the writer plenty of time. Even if he has plenty of time, however, the rate of writing will enter into the situation, because the child who writes slowly and labori-ously will be distracted by the mere process of writing and his recol-lection of ideas will be in a measure distracted by this mere process of setting down on paper what he has recalled. (Judd, 1914: 373)

A child whose writing is slow is likely to find their writing speed a barrier to recalling all the information they have gained from reading under examination. Slow writing under examination conditions may give the examiner the perception that a subject has a reading difficulty, when, in fact, their difficulty lies with their writing speed. The analytical dissection of the various attributes of reading and writing, and their subsequent examination, alerts educationalists to various aspects of these activities. This can allow for an understanding of how a precise difficulty with an aspect of reading, such as speed, could cause a child particular problems in the schoolroom. As the complexity of these processes is detailed, and knowledge of the potential difficulties that a student may encounter diffuses among professional and lay populations, the school and associated disciplines become more hospitable to the diagnosis. Congenital word-blindness therefore becomes a veritable diagnosis.

Waldo states that within the skill of reading there is great variation, with some children of lower grades being substantially better readers than their counterparts in higher grades (1915: 267). Waldo's recognition of a large variation in the abilities of the literate population illustrates that it has become technically possible to discern between various levels of reading ability among a school population. In turn, technological innovations in education facilitated the re-visualising of populations amongst the eager attempts to measure and record every difference that could be attributed to a body. Subsequently, the spectrum of reading ability was applied to the population.

William Gray (1916a), who, over the course of the next decade, published many articles on reading within the covers of *The Elementary School Journal*, in an article on the testing of reading ability, suggested that special attention should be attended to both pupils with higher and lower reading rates than the majority of the pupils. He then identifies a variety of reasons why a pupil may have a low reading rate:

> If some pupils are found who read at a rate much higher or lower than the majority of the class, special study should be made of these cases. The work may be too hard or too easy for them, they may have speech defects which need attention, their eyesight may be poor, they may have an unusually rapid rate of speaking which should be gradually reduced, or there may be other types of help of which they stand in need. Expert teaching and supervision involve the use of methods which will locate pupils who are in need of help. Objective tests are proving of great help in discovering such pupils. (1916a: 244)

Like Courtis (1914) and Judd (1914), Gray recognises the great utility of standard tests, as, for him, their usefulness relies upon their ability to discover pupils who will need specialist teaching methods to learn effectively. As a technology of government standard, tests are a tool of visualisation allowing for an individual or population to be seen in new ways, hence facilitating the more precise government of the educational population. Fast speech was suggested as an aetiological factor. This is something that was not encountered in the articles on congenital word-blindness reviewed in previous chapters. These technologies are deployed as a means of locating the pupils who are in the most need of attention, with expert teaching then directed towards them. These special cases are to be studied 'intensively', with the hope being that the specific barrier the subject is facing in their reading can be found and subsequent actions taken to eliminate it.

Understanding the text and speed of reading are once again separated and differentiated as different aspects of the skill of reading. The human body's abilities and attributes are being separated and segmented into smaller characteristics, allowing for the increasingly precise management of their abilities. As the diagram of human capabilities becomes more detailed, relations of power can flow in a more subtle manner. Gray (1916a) identifies that the level of understanding and the quality of the interpretation of a text is much harder to measure than the rate a child reads at:

> Reproduction and interpretation. The cultivation of the power to reproduce and understand is one of the important aims of most reading-exercises. This power differs greatly in different children, and is affected by the kinds of ideas presented in the reading-matter and by the quality of the teaching. It is more difficult to find out how much children understand and are able to reproduce than to determine the rate of reading. (1916a: 232)

These tests are to be understood as technologies that facilitate the re-imagining of a particular educational group. They transform bodies making a variety of differing abilities and characteristics visible, opening them to the activity of government. Gray discusses how

> A supervisor or principal may utilize the results of these tests in various ways. In oral reading the progress made by a given grade may be compared with the standard and an estimate made of the efficiency of the teaching for that grade. The relative achievement

of each pupil in the class may be determined. The dominant weaknesses of individuals and of classes are revealed by the original record of errors on the oral-reading sheets. The relative achievement of individuals and classes may be determined for speed and quality in silent reading. The figures reveal whether an individual or a class is weak primarily in speed or primarily in quality. The numbers representing the speed and quality for the individuals of a class may be compared to determine to what extent high speed favours good quality of reading. The question has probably arisen in the minds of many readers as to the reason for omitting the quality of expression, as well as various other points, from the method of testing oral reading. The fact that the quality of expression is omitted should not be construed as evidence that its value has been overlooked. Its omission from this scheme is due to the fact that no method has been devised as yet for testing the quality of expression in an impersonal way. It is recommended that each supervisor or teacher who gives oral-reading tests adopt a standard of judgment for himself and estimate the effectiveness of the expression of each pupil whom he tests, in addition to recording the other points outlined in the directions. The writer has followed this method in hundreds of cases with the result that a great deal of insight has been gained concerning the reading habits of pupils of different ages. The more one studies the problem of expression the more difficulties he finds in establishing a set of standards which would meet with common acceptance. (1916b: 298)

The results of a test are, of course, to be compared with the estimated standard for the grade. Working in assemblage with the norm, standard tests allowed for the generalisation of power from the individual body to the body of the population (Ewald, 1990: 141). The reading abilities of individuals, classes and entire schools can be analysed in this fashion. Tests can then be conducted to deduce to what extent speed favours good quality reading, providing information that allows for the construction of strategies for teaching those understood as having a difficulty with reading. Gray recognises that expression is the third attribute that should be considered when examining the schoolchildren's reading ability. It is noted that there is no way of studying this in an impersonal way, suggesting that a transposable method for measuring this skill had not been achieved. As this characteristic remained beyond the reach of these tools of measurement, it also remained beyond the reach of relations of power.

Teaching *Difficult* Readers

Clara Schmitt, author of the first article in a teaching journal concerned with congenital reading difficulties (Schmitt, 1914), had also devoted much of her article, 'School Subjects as Material for Tests of Mental Ability', to wider issues around reading. Schmitt considers the learning of reading to be the most important accomplishment in a child's school life (1914: 150–1). She states that the ability to acquire many other educational attributes is dependent upon the learning of this vital skill (a view shared by many of the writers discussed earlier who published in this journal). It is necessary that subjects learn to read so that their bodies are made amenable to the effects of technologies that enact more complex strategies of government. Therefore, many educational technologies rely upon a literate subject (again, as the papers discussed earlier described), as reading developed to be the major method by which instruction is given as a child progresses throughout their school life:

> The most important accomplishment in the school life is that of reading. The child's progress throughout the school is dependent entirely upon his attaining it. Upon it depends his progress, to a large extent, in arithmetic and almost entirely in history and geography and other such subjects which consist of classified or organized groups of facts. (Schmitt, 1914: 150–1)

The development of a certain standard of reading ability is considered to be the most important accomplishment in the child's schooling. A child's learning of geography, history or arithmetic is likely to be hampered if they cannot read printed texts. A specific difficulty with reading will thus prove problematic to almost every aspect of a child's education. By being imbued with the ability to read, the body becomes amenable to a whole variety of technologies of power. Literate bodies were necessary so that more specialised subject-based knowledge and skill could be cultivated in the aforementioned subjects.

Schmitt (1914) differentiates between two aspects of reading: 'quality' and 'quantity'. The activity of reading is thus being sectioned into two distinct skills. This splitting of the activity of reading resulted in the increasingly microscopic and multi-faceted visualisation of the individual body and the population (Ewald, 1991; Foucault, 1979; Hacking, 1982, 1990; Rose, 1999). This dissection of the activity of reading into smaller component parts took place because of a concern with cultivating better, efficient readers. This intent to cultivate more proficient readers, this attempt to establish more incisive technologies of government, made this distinction between 'quality' and 'quantity' in reading visible. The management of reading became concerned with such discrete attributes as those who read well, but slowly; those who could have techniques applied to them to improve their speed; and those who read quickly, but without quality. Once identified, these individuals could then have techniques and practices applied to them that would focus upon improving a specific attribute. This is an analogous process to the identification of reading difficulties by psychologists and ophthalmologists. In a feedback loop of sorts, psychologists' and ophthalmologists' work on reading difficulties provides evidence for the distinction between quality and quantity in reading, and this distinction makes reading difficulties an increasingly veritable diagnostic category. With further research into the process of reading taking place at an increasing rate, those who conducted studies into difficulties with reading had a large body of work to base such studies on. These studies developed the work done by others and in doing so added to the authoritative character of the research. By accepting the ideas found in these papers, educationalist's facilitated the flow of these ideas onto new sites and increased their professional acceptance. In short, reading difficulties became increasingly legitimate as detailed diagrams of different types of readers were drawn. Identifying that a deficient reader may be deficient in one or both of these aspects—quality or quantity—gave an extra dimension to the study of reading difficulties. Three types of congenital reading difficulties were now possible: those who were deficient in both aspects and those who were only deficient in one of them. Schmitt describes the different accomplishments that children's reading should be measured against in terms of quality and quantity:

> The accomplishment of the child in this subject may be arranged with reference to quantity and quality. A defective child may be deficient in one or both of these two characteristics of the reading accomplishment. He may be incapable of learning to recognize the words of the printed page; he may show himself capable of learning words only very slowly or of forgetting them quickly and easily. He may show himself capable of learning words with some facility in memorizing them, and so of becoming a good reader, but incapable of gaining ideas from the words which he reads. It is this latter characteristic which one is to understand as included in its various aspects under the term 'quality.' (1914: 151)

Schmitt's description of the process of learning to read illustrates that the ability of being able to acquire ideas from reading words, or the long term memorising of words learnt through reading, are the characteristics of quality reading. This is juxtaposed against quantity, wherein a reader is able to recognise a large number of words on the page, but is either unable to remember them in the long term or finds it harder to glean ideas from the process. Children can be defective in one or both of these processes. Sub-dividing the skill of reading into two disparate components allows for the increasing specialisation of technologies concerned with visualising populations. At the same time, it allows for the educational processes to be directed at smaller and distinct aspects of reading. This is one example of how the reach of strategies of government increased as technologies of power made complex diagrams of the individual body and the body of the population available. Segmenting the process of reading into two components allows a reader to be deficient in either or both. A difficulty with reading could now lie, for Schmitt (1914), wholly with the quality of reading or wholly with the quantity of reading. The segmentation of reading into various attributes allows for the strategy of fostering the ability to read among the body of the population to develop increasingly complex and precisely directed programmes involving intricate assemblages of technologies of power. They are calibrated to perform minute, but elaborate, operations upon those bodies that have been accredited with a reading difficulty. These involve difficulties with quantity. However, they are to managed by a different assemblage of technologies than difficulties with quality. In turn, a different assemblage of technologies would be applied to bodies that are understood as having difficulties with both these attributes.

A child who learns mainly through stimulus from the teacher is described by Schmitt (1914). They are therefore unable to learn new words from the printed page. This, of course, limits the speed at which the child can learn independently, resulting in a dramatic reduction in the general speed that a child can learn at. As independent study becomes an increasingly vital pedagogic device the further one progresses through the schooling system (Gray, 1919: 336). Schooling problematises the child accredited with a congenital reading difficulty as they are less receptive to the pedagogic methods deployed in later stages of schooling, where silent reading becomes increasingly prevalent in imparting information to students. The rate at which a student reads also becomes crucial as larger amounts of texts are to be consumed. While the child accredited as defective can be taught through stimulus provided by the teacher, it is apparent that this is more resource-intensive than reading texts themselves. Children accredited with reading difficulties are problematised because of the more resource-intensive character of their learning requirements.

Schmitt provides a description of the utilisation of the visual memory in children accredited as defective as a means for acquiring a vocabulary:

> The child may show an ability to recognize words from the printed page to a greater or less extent, but this recognition with the defective child consists, largely, merely of a mechanical type of visual memory which serves as a stimulus for its associated vocal prototype. The child who learns words in this way only is always dependent upon his teacher, since he can acquire for himself no new or unfamiliar word from the printed page. He can become somewhat independent of his teacher only if he learns phonetic values. Defective children are sometimes capable of acquiring very large visual vocabularies, but show themselves quite deficient in perceiving phonetic relationships. (1914: 151)

Phonetics here is identified as being the major stumbling block with which those readers accredited as defective encounter in their progress. Some children develop large 'visual' vocabularies, but their phonetic abilities were accredited as deficient in comparison. Vocabulary, like reading ability, is being segmented into distinct attributes. The segmentation of various abilities facilitated the cultivation of bodies by making it simpler to discern what attributes were in need of cultivation. Educational strategies, practices and technologies could then be developed that were concerned with fostering these. It is noted that it is rare that a child accredited as defective is encountered who is accomplished in phonetic problems. It was considered by Schmitt to be important that a student should become adept in the phonetic method of reading. This is because it would allow them to understand newly encountered words from their component parts and, in turn, develop relative independence from the teacher. Pupils equipped with the ability to work out new words on their own require less attention from the teacher, allowing for the pace of the acquisition of knowledge to augment, while the attention of the teacher can be diverted to other tasks. The problematisation of children who do not learn this method results not from their inability to perform a task but the speed at which they will perform it and the problems they engender for the distribution of a teacher's time. This level of comprehension and the subsequent stages are described by Schmitt:

Can read at sight any material such as newspaper, etc.: This is the highest grade which may be attained in the ability to read, with reference to quantity. It is attained by the normal child with the fifth grade. The phonetics which underlie the reading process is the great stumbling-block of the defective child. Seldom is one found who has this accomplishment. He may be able to learn a very few of the simplest combinations, such as consist of one or two consonants and a vowel. The normal child progresses in his knowledge of phonetic values to such an extent that he becomes independent of the teacher in so far as the illogical complexities of our English spelling permit. At the fourth grade the normal child is able to work out new and unfamiliar words with approximate phonetic correctness. (1914: 152)

Learning to read to this level allows children to become relatively autonomous in their education. Children in the USA, who have not achieved this level by the fourth grade, are classified as defective children unable to follow the normal child in deploying knowledge of phonetic values in their reading so that they become independent of their teacher. In contrast to the mechanical methods of reading that are typical of those children accredited as defective, Schmitt describes 'appreciative reading', a style of reading she believes is exhibited by the best readers; those who are able to dissect a text to show the most important parts and who often read with obvious pleasure and expression:

Appreciative: This type of reading is the opposite of the mechanical type just discussed. With this type there is usually expression of tone in reading which shows the child's understanding or appreciation of the selection read. Upon being questioned, he can tell in a sentence or more the essential elements of a selection. It is usually a sure sign that the reading has been appreciative if pleasure is shown. However, expression is not an infallible test. Defective children may be trained to read selections with expression, and if the circumstances of the training have been pleasant the child may incorporate these pleasant associations into the reading process itself, so that he seems to be enjoying the ideas derived from the selection. In such a case, however, he fails to read with expression or to reproduce the sense of the meaning when the same material is arranged in unfamiliar form. (1914: 154)

A discussion of reading with pleasure is utilised by Schmitt to imbue the activity of reading with positive associations. It is hoped that this will improve children accredited as having defective reading abilities. Schmitt suggests that the tone that a child uses while they are reading is often an indicator of their level of understanding. A further sign of appreciation is whether or not the subject has exhibited indications of pleasure in their tone:

> The reading of the defective children presents such irregular characteristics that averages which would present any meaning are difficult to obtain. The children tested had been much drilled in the story of the Fox and the Grapes. Nevertheless 24 of the 46 could read it with less facility than the first-grade children. They made many errors of the absurd type discussed above. Their reading consisted of some unerring recognition of words and more or less filling-in to supply a remembered context. Nine of the defectives could give only a scant account of the story and an incorrect interpretation. Twelve defective children were graded as equal to the first-grade child in reading ability. Ten were graded equal to the second-grade child in ability as regards the mechanical and qualitative aspects of the second reading test. Two of the defectives of the second grade could give an adequate account of the matter read. One of these children was ten years of age and by reason of this test and others was reclassified on his record sheet as only back-ward and returned to the regular grades of the school. The other, twelve years of age, was so deficient in other tests that he was retained in the special room. (1914: 161)

The child Schmitt considered the most deficient encountered difficulties that led to them being retained in the special room, evidencing that educational practices, following a logic of segregation were deployed in pronounced cases of reading difficulty. Segregating pupils according to their perceived abilities fits with the rationale of maximising the effective distribution of a teacher's time. Diagnostic categories like congenital word-blindness would facilitate the distributions of resources and skills onto bodies that required specific interventions. Standardised notions of the ability a child should have gained in a particular educational attribute, by a certain period, fabricate clear levels of attainment. If these are not achieved then the child would be perceived as falling behind or, perhaps, would be diagnosed with a particular impairment category. The importance of the standardisation of grades in the USA's education system is therefore apparent. The creation of this difference allowed the machinery of government concerned with education to operate on a microscopic level. The differences created by these standardised tests all required the norm to generalise disciplinary tactics of power onto a population (Ewald, 1991)

Four years after publishing her article on mental testing in the schoolroom, Schmitt returned to dealing with reading difficulties in school populations, writing two papers on congenital word-blindness (1918a, 1918b). These papers were important not only because they were the first papers dedicated to congenital word-blindness in educational journals but also because they detailed, for the first time, a programme for how the education of those accredited with congenital word-blindness was outlined. The papers were published in the *Elementary School Journal*, a periodical where a wide variety of papers concerned with reading and reading difficulties was published. Even though so many papers were published within these pages concerned with reading difficulties, alongside almost every other reading related issue, congenital word-blindness had not yet been written about. The significance of Schmitt's (1918a, 1918b) papers is that they mark the point that a particular technology of government moves from being discussed in strictly clinical sites to how the diagnosis may be utilised in relation to schooling.

While congenital word-blindness, alexia, visual deafness, amnesia visualis verbalis and dyslexia had, for some time now, been the preserve of medics, ophthalmologists or psychologists, from 1910 onwards teachers and educationalists begun to devote serious attention to all aspects of reading in their professional journals. Children who found learning to read difficult became a concern of these writers during this period. The pages of the *Elementary School Journal* reveal this to be the case, with numerous articles detailing a concern with all manner of the problematics of reading. Schmitt's 'Developmental Alexia: Congenital Word-Blindness, or Inability to Learn to Read', is the first time an educationalist considered how the diagnosis of congenital word-blindness would relate to the educational problematic. This develops out of her own earlier interest in reading difficulties (discussed earlier in this chapter) and the milieu of the journal (again, discussed earlier), where almost every imaginable aspect of reading was considered.

Thus far, psychologists who were concerned with congenital reading difficulties had aligned themselves with the discipline of clinical psychology, which, as previously discussed, had a clear educational remit. While the problem of congenital word-blindness had been discussed in academic journals previously, this was in the context of general concerns with a difficulty with reading. The move from a concern with reading difficulties in general to the operationalisation of technical devices generated in the medical and psychological communities, evidences the assembling of an array of apparatus for cultivating the development of children with specific difficulties within educational practice. The importation of a technology from medical and psychological communities to the educational environment signals the success of establishing a veritable diagnosis taken seriously by those not only in specialist networks but also in adjacent disciplines.

Schmitt's discussion begins with a definition of congenital word-blindness and a cursory reference to the deployment of dyslexia as an alternative title for the diagnosis:

> Congenital word-blindness, inability to learn to read, or dyslexia has been defined as an extreme difficulty to learn to recognize printed or written language on the part of persons otherwise normally endowed mentally and without defect of vision or other physical defect of such gravity as to constitute an interference of the process of learning to read. 'Congenital word-blindness' is the term used by nearly all writers on this condition and for that reason will be used throughout this report. (1918a: 680)

Congenital word-blindness is therefore considered not necessary as the clinically most appropriate term but, instead, as literary convention. The emphasis on the difficulty with reading being localised is again stated (as numerous previous papers have, and the definition is produced through reference to the diagram of the norm). While Schmitt states that congenital word-blindness will be used as it is the convention in the literature, she makes a concession to the advocates of the term developmental alexia in the titling of her paper. Although she provides references to both the psychological and the ophthalmological literature, the titling of her paper may suggest more of an affinity for the psychological over the ophthalmological literature, as here she chooses to deploy the term developmental alexia—a term associated with the University of Pennsylvania's psychological clinic (Witmer, 1916: 190).

Extensive diagnostic criteria are then provided, many of them exclusionary in their character. Some of these are health related and have not been seen thus far in the diagnostic criteria provided by the medical and psychological writers. Some pedagogical criteria are also stated. One of these educationally specific criteria is regular school attendance:

> These were found in a school population of 42,900 in fifty schools. The necessary conditions of such diagnosis are: (1) Regular school

attendance. (2) Reasonable good health and physical condition in general. No child showing evidence of poor nutrition, rachitis, much enlarged tonsils and adenoids, tuberculosis, kidney trouble, or other severe types of physical disability should be so diagnosed. (3) No sign of visual defect. (4) Pre-existing extreme slowness in learning to read; or total inability, manifested over one or more years of school life. (5) General mental ability good or average. (6) No other interfering factor, such as foreign language in the home, dislike of school, abnormal unresponsiveness to school or other social situations, etc. There are many cases of slowness in learning to read which are complicated by one or more of the contributing factors above. Learning to read is an exceedingly complex process requiring continuity and concentration of attention. Therefore any weakening of the physical condition interferes with the process and causes backwardness in the attainment of facility in reading to a much greater extent than other subjects are affected granted that there is not innate mental defect. (1918a: 686)

This extensive list of other physical criteria is utilised to eliminate the possibility that the characteristics associated with congenital word-blindness are not being caused by anything else. Reading is to be understood as an 'exceedingly complex process'. Factors, whether they be social or biological, that could put the diagnosis' veritable character in doubt were to be excluded. These included various health conditions (tuberculosis, kidney trouble) and visual impairments. Social factors, such as good school attendance, generally good physical and mental health, and foreign languages being spoken at home, were to be excluded. Hinshelwood (1907) had attempted to protect the diagnosis fearing sceptics looking for reasons to dismiss the diagnostic category. Schmitt continues this practice.

The necessity of none of these factors being present to confidently make the diagnosis allows congenital word-blindness to operate as a precise tool of differentiation, a technology for marking and organising bodies. A parallel should again be drawn to the concerns of Hinshelwood detailed in Chapter 4. The extensive lists of criteria exacerbate the function (discussed in Chapters 4 and 5) of distinguishing those diagnosed with congenital word-blindness from the feeble-minded, or those with a reading difficulty and a more general failing of intelligence. The potency of the function of the diagnosis continues to be one of the paramount concerns of those writing on word-blindness. Schmitt's concern with maintaining, or, indeed, increasing the potency of the function and the veritable character of the diagnosis lead her to suggest some criteria that would make it difficult for anybody to ever be diagnosed as congenitally word-blind, such as there being no previous interfering difficulty in reading.

Mental examinations were to be deployed as the method for ascertaining whether the patient can be considered to be congenitally word-blind: 'The examination of the children here reported consists of a physical and mental examination' (Schmitt, 1918a: 686). A convention was established to obtain 'a report of health and developmental history wherever possible' (ibid). Hereditary information has established itself as a necessary and important part of reviewing a patient's history and making a diagnosis in tandem with the employment of various tests and devices for measuring particular attributes. Schmitt advocates the use of intelligence tests. However, the traditional intelligence test produced by Binet and Terman is treated as a flawed tool in the diagnosis of word-blindness. Schmitt advocates the deployment of the test she developed in her paper 'Standardization of Tests for Defective Children', and details her reasons for considering them problematic:

In the mental examination those tests are most relied upon which show the child's ability to think or reason. It is the practice of the writer to use such tests for innate intelligence as depend least upon experience or teaching which cannot or may not easily be evaluated by the examiner. In the examinations for mental ability of the general public-school clinic one cannot depend slavishly upon scales of measurement of mental age, however excellently these may have been constructed with reference to the average child and his experiences. The problem child is more or less outside the experiences usual to the child who is in all respects normal and must be examined and diagnosed always with reference to this possibility. It is not the writer's practice to determine a 'mental age' in every case. The time to do this is added to the ordinary examination only occasionally. Some of the tests which enter into the various scales for determining mental ability are always used, for the most part those testing reasoning ability. The writer's attitude toward tests of mental ability was (Schmitt 1918: 687) discussed to some extent in the monograph, 'Standardization of Tests for Defective Children.' The writer can only apologize to the readers of this article who are accustomed to think of mental ability in terms of the mental age of some one of the scales for its measurement, but they can be assured that enough of the Binet and Terman scales were given in all but two cases to assure an approximate normal mental age, though a definite statement of a mental age in months cannot be made from the tests given. The thought of publication of results came only after the usual procedure for determining mental ability and a diagnosis of the cause of the child's trouble had been made for some time. Then, too, the data are the result of a gradual accumulation and were not obtained as one whole and connected problem but garnered out of the mass of all cases seen. (1918a: 688)

Details of how the author proceeds with her modified mental examinations for children suspected of being congenitally word-blind are given (they are also further elaborated in her 1915 article, 'Standardization of Tests for Defective Children'). In the literature that has been discussed in the preceding chapters, the tests deployed have not been systematically laid out, and the Binet test and Terman scale were frequently deployed. Schmitt's modified intelligence tests utilise personal information about the subject, arithmetic, spelling, shape and colour work:

The mental examination is made along the following lines: First, by way of becoming acquainted with the child's general traits of responsiveness, social orientation, use of language, and to give him time to get on a friendly footing with the examiner he is asked about age, birthday, place of abode, father's occupation, number of brothers and sisters, their ages, grades in school, what they are doing now, etc. Children who know such family data are always glad to tell it. Any spontaneousness or volunteer information is encouraged with a show of interest that the child may feel free in expressing himself. (1918a: 688)

This general discussion aims to put the child at ease and gain a sense of the child's competence with language, social interaction and conversation. Achieving a friendly footing with the examiner is necessary so that the child performs to his/her best potential throughout the rest of the test. Encouraging spontaneousness develops a rapport with the child, and may give the examiner information about his/her character. The test then moves onto examining the child's abilities with mathematics:

Secondly, he is given school tests of reading, arithmetic, etc. A child's comprehension of arithmetic and his ability to deal with arithmetical problems is an important bit of evidence in making a diagnosis of mental ability. Many high-grade defective children learn arithmetical processes without the ability to use the same in thinking ways or to comprehend the mathematical meaning of what they have learned. A child may have learned the process of long division, for instance, without being able to find the solution of such a problem as, If 5 pencils cost 10 cents, how much will you have to pay for one pencil ? He may by some accident of school life not have learned the processes of work with fractions taught in the fifth grade, but he may possess an understanding of the arithmetical meaning of fractions and do problems in reasoning with fractional parts not involving the knowledge of book processes. The child who has learned arithmetic in normal fashion has shown his ability to think of abstract concepts in symbolic terms. The ability to use symbols to represent abstract conceptions is the most significant distinguishing characteristic of the normal human mind of our civilization. (1918a: 688–9)

Schmitt's insistence on the ability to interpret symbols to understand abstract notions is a distinguishing feature between the 'normal human of our civilization' and those whom she accredited as defective in some fashion. This is a conceptual formulation that is not deployed by any of the writers I have discussed in this book. Hinshelwood (1896: 1508) had previously argued that children accredited with congenital word-blindness are often able to read figures despite their difficulty reading other written symbols. The addition of a variance in how subjects learn mathematics, and the large emphasis placed upon this, is an innovation that separates Schmitt's work from much that had come before it. Schmitt is offering a recalibrated version of the diagnosis.

Reading and related skills are the next set of attributes that Schmitt examines:

In the reading tests one learns just how much the child can read, how well he can handle phonics as an aid in reading new or unfamiliar material, whether he gets information from reading, and whether he can organize the material read by giving a full account or an adequate account of it with the omission of only unnecessary details. With the children who cannot read their ability to make the perceptual discriminations necessary is tested by asking them to match words. For this test page 103 of the Howe First Reader is used. On this page many words are repeated several times throughout the selection. The examiner points to any one of the words the child does not know and asks him to find another just like it on the page. He is given all the time necessary to find it. A circle is drawn about the sample word to help him in finding it again for comparison with the words he thinks may fit the requirements. He is given several such until the examiner is certain he does or does not possess such powers of discrimination. On the same page in juxtaposition are the words 'our' and 'out.' The child is asked to look carefully and say whether the words are exactly alike, and when he reports that they are not to point out with the pencil the parts that are different. (1918a: 689)

In addition to the deployment of tests and devices of her own making, in this examination Schmitt uses the 'test found on page 103 of the Howe First Reader'. Various skills are tested by her, such as the ability to distinguish between very similar words, match up the same word, find synonyms and glean information from a text. These tests are utilised in assemblage to produce a precise diagram of the character of the difficulty with reading the subject is encountering. Various other devices are then deployed 'for the purpose of giving expression to thinking ability are' (Schmitt, 1918a: 690):

the counting backward test, the difference test of the Binet Scale, the likeness tests of the Terman Scale, the puzzle tests one, three, and four of the Healy-Fernald Series, the cross-lines A and B of the same series, a time orientation test, opposites test, the Healy pictorial completion test, etc. This is almost a minimum list for young children which is extended downward or upward with reference to the particular problem of the particular child under examination. To some children a test of colour analysis is given. This test is possible because the colour grey is not; commonly taught in the first grade and many children do not know it. They sometimes hazard the names black or white, but readily agree that it is not like the black or white shown them. They are then asked to make a name for it and often they decide to call it a faded or light black or a dark or dirty white. (1918a: 689–90)

In the time orientation test, children of first- and second-grade age are not penalized if they do not know the names of the days of the week. They are graded satisfactory if they know that the current day is not Sunday, and say in answer to stimulating questions that it is a week day or a school day and can tell what they do on Saturday and Sunday. The time test can be made more and more complex for older children until it involves historical data. The memory tests commonly used are digits heard and the two Binet designs. For other evidence teachers are questioned concerning the child's school reactions, his ability with the handwork of the school, apathy or diligence in work, etc. In the following accounts of cases the attempt is made to describe the child's intelligence in terms of a few of his highest reactions and whatever his disabilities may be in terms of his lowest reactions, rather than to take the necessary space to describe the mental examination in detail. The children here reported showed up normal with respect to the various lines of inquiry mentioned above unless otherwise stated. (1918a: 690)

This description of how a test to ascertain whether a child can be diagnosed as congenitally word-blind details the different tests that were used to examine various different mental faculties. All aspects of the child's intelligence have to be tested, as congenital word-blindness is considered to be a localised condition, only affecting the part of the brain concerned with reading. Therefore, the child has to be passed as normal in all other areas. These tests are part of the machinery of government that allows for the localisation of the difficulty to be guaranteed. *The Howe First Reader* is referred to as a technology for testing some attributes of children who may be congenitally word-blind.

Schmitt's paper was published in two parts. The first part was discussed earlier in this chapter and concentrated on Schmitt's technical suggestion regarding the testing process. The second part is a more conventional discussion of three case studies. Schmitt's paper is noteworthy for two reasons: (1) it is the first paper dealing exclusively with word-blindness to be published in an educational journal; (2) it is the first case of several cases occurring in the same school. Owing to this latter reason, Schmitt proposes some specific methodologies for teaching word-blind children in groups, incorporating techniques that had, at this point, not been explored.

Cases 9, 10, 11, and 12, were placed in a special room with a teacher who had given special attention to methods of teaching reading. This placement was possible because all these children were found in the same school. In no other instance was more than one such child found in a school, and it was not considered expedient to place the child with subnormal children. In these cases it was felt that no injustice would be done, since a large part of the members of the room were not definitely subnormal, but backward for a variety of reasons.

Some of the backward ones were as poor in reading as the subjects of this article, but from physical or other causes. (1918b: 757)

The finding of multiple cases in one school iterates that the rarity of the condition was being called into question, not only discursively, but also by the number of examples occurring at a single site. These subjects were to be educated together, separating them from the normal school population. Schmitt, however, perceives it as unjust to place these children with children she refers to as 'sub-normal'; children accredited as congenitally word-blind undergo a process of differentiation from both those children accredited as normal and subnormal. Schmitt attempts to differentiate the children accredited with congenital word-blindness from the children in the 'special room' and the other inhabitants of this room, the 'sub-normal'. The distinction here between backward and subnormal is intriguing as being sub-normal is seemingly, for Schmitt, more problematic than being accredited as backward. Being understood as belonging to these different groups appears to imbue a body with different moral values.

The biological and inherited image of specific reading difficulties is affirmed, as already encountered in Thomas (1905), Stephenson (1907) and Hinshelwood (1907), and the well-trodden path that children accredited with word-blindness may still be able to read figures is reiterated (Hinshelwood, 1896). Schmitt refers to a variety of different aetiologies for congenital word-blindness that has been described by various writers:

The cause assigned by most writers indicates a lesion in brain structure and is termed variously, 'biologic variation,' 'phenomenon of atavism,' 'lack of development of left angular gyrus.' Rieger assigns the condition to the field of general intelligence; Voss's free association experiment and Jackson's discussion suggest the same. Among those who entertain the idea of lesion of the reading center some have assigned the recognition of figures and musical characters to different centers than that for reading, since most congenital word-blind cases can recognize one or both of these types of symbols. (1918b: 765)

Aetiologies grounded in a brain centre lesion are questioned by Schmitt owing to the achievements of children who received special instruction in reading:

In the light of the reading ability developed by the children who received special teaching, one must doubt the theory of a specialized brain center lesion. We must assume in case of the lesion theory that, in the brain of the congenital word-blind child who has learned to read, connections with some other group of brain cells has been made by the stimulus-receiving center involved and that the new center then took over the specialized function of storing word images, a conception not in line with the trend of current thought concerning imagery; or that the center biologically set aside for this purpose has undergone a development of some sort. The latter is, of course, untenable. (1918b: 765)

Schmitt suggests that the evidence of children accredited with congenital word-blindness learning to read and contemporaneous research into the brain disproves the lesion theories that had been put forward by Hinshelwood (1896, 1990b, 1902, 1907). In opposition to these biological aetiologies, which were often based on lesions, and had been the mainstream in the literature, Schmitt chooses to affirm a psychological aetiology: 'This failure on the part of a child who is otherwise normal may be related to the psychology of meaning and association' (1918b: 766). Congenital word-blindness is iterated as being a condition of childhood where the subject is in all other ways, apart from their localised difficulty with the lexicon, understood to be normal. The proposal of an aetiology resulting from a failure of meaning and association is Schmitt's own innovation: the diagram of reading abilities becomes more complex still. Schmitt considers meaning to be composed of various factors and experiences:

> We know that the complex which goes to make up that mental quality termed 'meaning' and associated with all precepts is composed of the many factors of experience in connection with the particular percept. It is made up of memories of smell, taste, colour, tactual qualities, kinaesthetic experiences, relations to other objects of perception, etc. Along with these experiences and knitting them into a functional whole are the ideas of the individual's past and present purposes with reference to the object of perception. When a certain such complex has been repeated in its entirety many times it is probable that in many instances a mental set or attitude is formed and, becoming habitual, may be closed to the admission of additional factors whose addition would make necessary a reconstruction of the percept complex and the formation of a new attitude. This is commonly known to be the case with complex motor processes. A person who has formed a certain motor habit can only with difficulty or not

at all reconstruct it, as witness inefficient golf, typewriting, hand-writing, piano playing, etc. (1918b: 766)

It is proposed that through an individual's experiences with a complex motor process, it can become incredibly difficult to reconstruct the pro-cess as it is related to various types of memory. Difficulties in specific areas are posited as most likely being habitual. Schmitt makes the asser-tion that '[t]he children who exhibit the characteristics of congenital word-blindness have minds which have become set in certain respects' (1918b: 767). This difficulty is not considered to necessarily affect all symbols: 'They may not be set in all such ways as would eliminate all printed language. This is shown by the fact that in nearly all cases reported there was ability to recognize figures and in some ability to read music' (Schmitt, 1918b: 767). This follows ground familiar to early cases of aphasia: acquired word-blindness (Broadbent, 1872; Hinshelwood, 1895; Kussmaul, 1877) and congenital word-blindness (Hinshelwood, 1900b; Morgan, 1896). The theory that Schmitt (1918b) posits to explain the tendency for subjects accredited with congenital word-blindness to being able to interpret other symbols, is distinct amongst the papers I have reviewed, and again relies upon the notion of habit:

The explanation for this is that there were few or no experiences with numbers and music before the symbols were presented and therefore no habit percept formed. The printed symbols of such sub-jects is, with most children, presented along with the child's other experiences with the subject-matter and thus are made a part of the habit percept complex. One case reported learned to read Latin read-ily while still finding much difficulty with English. This case may be explained in the same way. Latin words and their printed symbols went to form a new percept and did not necessitate the rearrange-ment of old ones. For the same reason Case 2 learned to read material in connection with his electrical work. (1918b: 767)

The psychological aetiology being expounded suggests that specific reading difficulties are essentially engendered by the development of what is considered to be a flawed motor habit. Schmitt elaborates on this explanation by suggesting that this motor habit is typically encountered as:

These same children fail to learn the phonics necessary to the read-ing process because the already-formed speech motor habits have never been subjected to such processes of synthetic analysis as accompanies the learning of phonics and have never consciously been applied to such uses. (1918b: 767)

A relation between the incorrect leaning of phonics and a difficulty with reading is suggested by Schmitt (1914). In Schmitt's hands congenital word-blindness has been transformed from a neurobiological diagnosis to a psychological diagnosis; its aetiology, for Schmitt (1918b), rests in a developmental process, rather than a subject's biology and its family history.

Remedial Reading

Between the covers of the *Elementary School Journal*, the wider problem of reading difficulties was investigated under the banner of remedial reading. The articles I will now discuss follow Schmitt's work, but do not utilise the vocabularies of either the ophthalmologists or the psychologists whom I have previously discussed. Instead, I shall situate these investigations under the more general banner of remedial reading. These articles show how educational sites were becoming increasingly hospitable to the problematic of congenital reading difficulties that had been raised in journals of ophthalmology and psychology. C. J. Anderson and Elda Merton's three-part article (1920a, 1920b, 1921) on remedial reading criticises the methods of the mass instruction of reading: 'Much of the weakness in our methods of teaching reading is due to our system of mass instruction which does not attempt to discover the sources of the reading ailments of individuals' (1920a: 685). The need to understand the individual difficulties with reading and establish methods for overcoming a variety of different difficulties with reading is identified. Anderson and Merton split so-called defects in those concerned with 'oral- and silent-reading' (1920a: 685). A move is then made to segment them further, again across the aspects of quality, comprehension and speed (Anderson and Merton, 1920a: 685).

The cases presented by Anderson and Merton across this three-part article have difficulties with reading for a wide variety of reasons. Case 'A' is able to read symbols and words far beyond her comprehension (1920a: 687–9). Case 'B' seems the most similar to cases diagnosed as having congenital word-blindness, and I shall therefore be giving a fuller description later (1920a: 692–3). Case 'C' is identified as lacking the necessary phonetic knowledge to develop her reading skills; the description refers to Case 'B' and marks their similarities. It is suggested that many of the same techniques of instruction were deployed as in Case 'C' (1920b: 772). Case 'D' is a boy who is, perhaps, closest to the interests of researchers concerned with congenital word-blindness, as his reading is lower than his achievements in other grades, and his physical examination and attendance records identify no reason why his reading would be falling behind his other grades (1920b: 778). Case 'E' describes a child where English is not spoken as a first language at home, thus resulting in a limited vocabulary, and where defective hearing and large-scale absence from school is found (1920b: 783). Case 'F' is a boy who is described as having a background that is not conducive to learning and whose parents have no time to take an interest in his education (1920b: 785). Anderson and Merton's interests are with reading difficulties in the broadest sense, but they are concerned with distinguishing between different types of difficulties, as different types of difficulties will require distinct techniques to be deployed to improve the subject's reading.

The description of Case 'B' is similar to the positive descriptions that I described in cases of congenital word-blindness provided by Hinshelwood (1900a, 1902, 1907), Nettleship (1901) and Thomas (1905). 'He has intelligent American foster parents and his home environment is good. He is exceedingly active on the playground and talks intelligently when asked questions (Anderson and Merton, 1920a: 693). Reports from his teacher indicate that he was considered to have excellent health and conduct—the elimination of other possible aetiologies that have been encountered in Hinshelwood. Schmitt and Witmer's work is again deployed. A brief description of the character of the boy's difficulty with reading identifies its similarity to cases of congenital word-blindness: 'Before training, his span of recognition was never more than a word and that word was seldom correctly given. He was unable to get anything out of silent reading, because he did not know his words' (Anderson and Merton, 1920a: 683).

Specialist individual training was positioned as being a successful methodology to improve readers who were not responding well to the homogenous character of reading instruction. With Case 'B', reading grades improved after a month of specialist training (Anderson and Merton, 1920a: 683), although previously they had not been able to achieve over a grade 'C' in second grade reading work. Anderson and Merton's attempt to individualise classroom teaching in reading, 'so that the pupils could be given remedial treatment according to their particular needs' (Anderson and Merton, 1921: 336), should be understood as symptomatic of technologies of government becoming increasingly microscopic, focusing on the individual body, while trying to cultivate a population. Both the general concern with reading difficulties that is found in Anderson and Merton (1920a, 1920b, 1921), and their attempts to segment this wider problematic in different areas describing specific problems, suggests that, at least for some writers, education was becoming a more hospitable site for the deployment of a diagnosis such as congenital word-blindness. The suggestions provided by Anderson and Merton for teaching children accredited as remedial illustrate that a diagnosis such as congenital word-blindness would facilitate the education of some of the children they described as remedial. This was of particular use to strategies of government concerned with capitalising the population.

Conclusion

In this chapter I have attempted to describe some of the texts that indicate that both educational experts and the site of the school were becoming increasingly hospitable to the diagnosis congenital word-blindness. I described how educationalists venerated the act of reading, understanding this to be a remarkably important characteristic (Bowden, 1911; Gray, 1919: 334; Guilfoile, 1921); believing it to foster the development of imagination; giving students the ability to learn more complex knowledge or specialist skills as they progress through school; and equipping students with the ability to learn independently from their teachers (Schmitt, 1914: 151). Literacy became an obligatory attribute that all children had to acquire during their schooling. It was necessary to imbue bodies with the ability to read if more complex skills were going to be able to be fostered during their education. Learning to read imbues bodies with the ability to learn independently. A difficulty with reading would therefore be an extremely problematic characteristic for strategies of government concerned with fostering individuality. A literate body, with the ability to learn independently, could be articulated into the activity of sculpting itself into the type of body that strategies of government desired the population to be filled with. I have argued that the numerical plotting of the population, as described in Chapter 2, facilitated the measuring of a subject's ability to read. More specifically, these technologies worked in assemblage with the norm, describing increasingly specific attributes of intelligence, and comparing them with standards that had been deduced to be normal. Various tests and procedures contributed to the modelling of a diagram of the activity of reading and various types of readers. Variance in how people read could now be visualised and acted upon. Schmitt (1918a, 1918b) provides an account of how the teaching of reading to children accredited with congenital word-blindness could proceed. Schmitt's proposition of a psychological aetiology suggests that educationalists found these explanations for congenital reading difficulties more persuasive than the accounts provided by the British ophthalmologists.

It is evident that the rationales of educating populations placed significant importance upon the production of literate bodies. An array of techniques and technologies were produced to make sure that as many bodies as possible achieved this obligatory point. Anderson and Merton (1920a, 1920b, 1921) opposed the homogenised character of the teaching of literacy. Instead, they proposed methods of sub-dividing the teaching of reading, developing techniques that were directed to improve different aspects of the skills of reading printed symbols. Among educationalists, reading itself was coming to be understood as having different characters. As such, it was argued that methods should be found to teach children with variant strands of reading difficulties. The discursive formations that coagulated around education in the 1920s became increasingly hospitable to the possibility of congenital reading difficulties.

8
Conclusion

I have argued that the formation of the diagnostic category dyslexia was not just the invention of a psycho-medical category, but also the invention of a technology of power. This technology was then deployed in assemblage with a variety of other technologies, such as the norm, intelligence tests, medical examinations and many others, as part of a machinery of government intended to perform minute and intricate operations. In the preceding discussion I have described the formation and solidification of the diagnosis that would become dyslexia. I have outlined the various different operations it performed in the hands of writers such as Hinshelwood (1895), Thomas (1905), Witmer (1907a, 1907b) and Rutherford (1909). The discussion that follows summarises the main arguments of the book, establishes the historical and theoretical contributions it has made, argues for the importance of producing other genealogies of impairment categories and makes some speculative remarks about the character of reading in the twenty-first century.

The Fashioning of Congenital Word-blindness and the Establishment of a Jurisdiction

The field of congenital reading difficulties was initially formed out of studies of aphasic patients who had lost the ability to read as a result of brain injury. Losing the ability to read owing to an injury was initially under the jurisdiction of medicine, considered to be one of an array of aphasias as seen in such work as Broadbent (1872) and Kussmaul (1877). Patients with these characteristics were often brought to the surgeries of ophthalmologists because of the perception of their difficulty with reading having an ocular origin. Ophthalmologists established their own diagnostic category—acquired word-blindness—and developed a relatively firm jurisdiction over these characteristics. Their diagnostic category, however, was still reliant upon a diagram of the brain that had been produced by Broadbent in his 1872 paper. Yet the necessity of this diagnosis was constituted by patients with these characteristics being brought to the surgeries of ophthalmologists. Like aphasia it was concerned with individuals who had lost, in this case, the ability to read. It was therefore concerned with individuals rather than populations.

It became possible to diagnose congenital reading difficulties in the 1890s as a result of three key factors coalescing: acquired word-blindness providing the technological foundations for the diagnosis; the introduction of mass schooling in the UK; and the affect that a style of government shifting towards bio-politics had on the practice of medicine, which became articulated into the activity of producing populations. The proliferation of this diagnostic category into the toolkit of ophthalmologists spread the diagram of the brain that Broadbent (1872) had developed. This gave ophthalmologists access to a particular assemblage of technologies that allowed for a particular population, brought to their surgeries, to be understood anew. In these surgeries a diagnosis was crafted to describe the characteristics that are today explained as dyslexia; it was named congenital word-blindness. This marked a shift from considering individuals accredited as defective, to being able to understand populations as defective. Rose has documented a similar move in psychology (1984: 161). Children who had pronounced difficulties with reading, despite their obvious intelligence, were brought to be examined by ophthalmologists. These difficulties made it hard for them to continue with their studies. The category of acquired word-blindness was thus recalibrated by the British ophthalmologists, and a technology for diagnosing these children was produced.

The problematic surrounding congenital reading difficulties found its initial expression as congenital word-blindness, a diagnosis initially associated with British ophthalmologists—a problematic that was formed after education became compulsory in 1870. These children were problematised because, despite their perceived intelligence, they were not responding to the techniques of education. I have illustrated how education was part of a bio-political style of governing concerned with the capitalisation of the population. The operation of congenital word-blindness is a response to the character of a bio-politics concerned with distilling worth from bodies previously understood to be worthless. I have argued that socio-economic factors, such as the move towards an economy increasingly characterised by cognitive labour, the proliferation of *l'homme moyen*, the rise of individual psychology, the articulation of medicine into the activity of statecraft and the introduction of mass education were all related to the formation of the diagnosis. My analysis has, however, suggested that all of these factors can be seen as part of a shift in the style of government away from sovereign power, towards bio-politics—a style of government where the population is understood as capital. I have therefore argued that the operation that congenital word-blindness performs as a technology of power is bio-political.

Hinshelwood's diagnosis of congenital word-blindness performed the operation of distinguishing those diagnosed with a congenital reading difficulty from those accredited as normal or feeble-minded; the diagnosis operated as a filter, enacting a process of differentiation between bodies initially understood as belonging to the wider population of those accredited as feeble-minded. This filtering process separated those who had a localised difficulty with reading from those who were accredited as having more pronounced difficulties with learning. Differences were also established between those bodies, which, through the precise application of an assemblage of technologies of power (that among other things included the norm, intelligence tests and educational practices), could overcome or minimise their accredited difficulties with reading, and those that could not. Congenital word-blindness illustrated that these bodies could have more worth drawn from them. The development of increasingly microscopic ways of conceiving of human characteristics, such as congenital word-blindness, facilitated the microscopic government of the body and the population. Rehabilitating these bodies was a means of harnessing increased capital from the workforce. This perpetuated both the rationality of education as a social good, benefiting both the state and those individuals now deemed to be worthy workers. No doubt the professionalisation of medicine and their articulation into the activity of statecraft described by Osborne (1993, 1997) moved the disciplines focus from the study of individuals accredited as defective to populations accredited as defective. What is peculiar here is that ophthalmologists were at the forefront of establishing this technology. Despite being eye specialists, ophthalmologists had been articulated into the government of educational difference. Congenital word-blindness was a technology able to achieve the goals of cultivating a population by operating on a microscopic element of an individual, an attribute of their intelligence. A diagnosis that concentrated on localised learning difficulties, seemingly microscopic elements of an individual, suggests that the diagram of the human that power is able to operate upon is no longer limited by what is immediately perceivable to the five human senses.

Various different diagnoses concerned with congenital reading difficulties were proposed by physicians and, more specifically, other ophthalmologists. In the USA, Rutherford's (1909) diagnosis performed a negative function, inscribing negative connotations, such as being defective or hopeless, onto bodies. In contrast, Hinshelwood's version of the diagnosis imbued the value of deservingness onto the bodies it accredited. While Hinshelwood and his associates' (Thomas, 1905) version of the diagnosis achieved relative dominance in the first decades of the twentieth century, the challenges continually made to them by ophthalmologists in the USA and Germany undermined its institutionalisation. This illustrates how different medical groups were utilising different versions of the diagnosis. I have argued that the differences between Rutherford's and Hinshelwood's version of the diagnosis are, perhaps, related to the ways that eugenics differed in the two countries, and how this resulted in the two countries having distinct styles of bio-politics. While the problem of congenital reading difficulties had been bought to prominence by the ophthalmologists, they were unable to maintain a jurisdiction over it. During the first decades of the twentieth century, psychology's prominence was rapidly growing on both sides of the Atlantic. Psychologists were thus able to establish a dominance over the problem of congenital reading difficulties, challenging the authority of the ophthalmologists, whose influenced had waned by the 1920s.

When the University of Pennsylvania's Psychological Clinic came under the leadership of Witmer, congenital reading difficulties became one of its central concerns, as seen in the founding documents of the Psychological Clinic's journal (Witmer, 1907a). Congenital reading difficulties were written about several times in the early years of *The Psychological Clinic*, and the tone of these article was noticeably different those of the ophthalmologists. The differing tone of American and British bio-politics was one of the factors that led to the diagnosis performing a different operation in *The Psychological Clinic* than in the hands of British ophthalmologists. While Hinshelwood and the British ophthalmologists had been concerned with emphasising the deserving character of the children they diagnosed with congenital word-blindness, they were also anxious to limit the number of bodies that the diagnosis could be applied to. This was motivated by a concern with maintaining the potency of its operation. The writers associated with the psychological clinic, however, were happy to apply this diagnosis to a wider variety of the population. The diagnosis was even attached to college students who had not encountered any educational difficulties in their previous schooling. The writers associated with *The Psychological*

Clinic were concerned with promoting the unproblematic quality of the characteristics, comparing congenital reading difficulties to being left-handed or not being able to sing in tune. This was, perhaps, because the eugenics movement in the USA was concerned with the elimination of negative characteristics. As I have described, when in the hands of Rutherford (1909) the characteristics that congenital word-blindness described became understood as negative. In this fashion Witmer, Ford and Town's framing of visual deafness, amnesia visualis verbalis and congenital word-blindness stopped it from being deployed in a machinery of government that was concerned with achieving negative eugenic programmes. This led to the diagnosis being concerned with the management of characteristics that were considered to be of an unproblematic kind; the methods that Witmer, Ford and Town suggested should be deployed were similar to those that Hinshelwood had advocated being deployed onto the bodies with pronounced characteristics. This illustrates the intensifying reach of machineries of government concerned with capitalising the population, and the increasing need to manage slight deviations from the norm. In the hands of Witmer, Town and Ford, amenisa visualis verbalis, and, later, congenital word-blindness, performed an increasingly minute operation. I would argue that this was because in the context of American bio-politics, negative eugenics had made the category of 'unproblematic difference' smaller than it was in the UK. The Psychological Clinic's diagnosis was concerned with drawing increased worth not from bodies that were considered to be worthless but from bodies that were already considered to have some worth. It operated to further capitalise an already capitalised population.

The child, as Rose has described (1984), provided the central axis upon which the formation and institutionalisation of individual psychology occurred. I have also described above how the researchers at the University of Pennsylvania's Psychological Clinic actively fostered relations with schools and other educational institutions, positioning the child accredited as defective as an object under their rubric of concern. Two important points are to be drawn from this. First, as psychology was formed, the discipline had an ever increasing array of diagnoses that could be applied to the bodies of children. As the discipline's prominence grew, the other technologies that the diagnosis relied upon (intelligence tests, standardised reading tests, conceptions of the norm relating to the mind) were increasingly related to psychology as well. The second point to be considered here is that the University of Pennsylvania's Psychological Clinic was actively concerned with fostering links with educational institutions, and was successful in doing so, thus dispersing their version of the diagnosis category directly into schools. This allowed for psychology to develop a jurisdiction over congenital reading difficulties, as psychology's distinction over the child accredited as defective augmented, while ophthalmology's hold over the problematic of congenital reading difficulties weakened. This positioned psychologists as better able to constitute an effective machinery of government than ophthalmologists.

Across the book I have argued that as part of the capitalisation of the population, at the end of the nineteenth and the beginning of the twentieth century, it became obligatory to be able to read to a certain standard. Having a difficulty with reading became problematic; as the British economy became increasingly specialised jobs required a higher degree of literacy. This is evidenced by the rise of the individual, the professions, the middle classes and the moves towards an economy increasingly characterised by cognitive labour. The strategy of proliferating reading throughout the body of the population was thus entwined with a bio-politics that was concerned with individualising bodies, imbuing them with the skills and the values of the middle classes, what Davis called *l'homme moyen*. As the acuteness of the characteristics that needed to be present for a diagnosis to be made decreased in their severity, congenital word-blindness began to perform a more minute operation. As a technology of power, congenital word-blindness facilitated an increasingly microscopic bio-politics. A bio-politics that was increasingly microscopic in the sense that it focused on drawing value from smaller more discrete characteristics. The Psychological Clinic of the University of Pennsylvania transformed congenital word-blindness into a diagnosis that performed the operation of further capitalising populations that were already capitalised.

In Witmer's work, *amnesia visualis verbalis* is constituted as a precise difference from the norm. Crucially, it was also constituted as a non-problematic variation, with comparisons made to being left-handed or not being able to sing in tune. The diagnosis followed a trajectory that took it from the most pronounced of cases, where the differentiation process had to be vociferous, and was achieved through a colourful description of the extremity of the intelligence of the subjects in question, to a quieter, more minute, yet more sophisticated, process. The characteristics that are being diagnosed were described as being an unproblematic difference, compared, for instance, with left-handedness, but they were, nonetheless, a difference that should be strived to be corrected. The operation of congenital word-blindness was precise and discrete, concerned with identifying and then correcting what was in some cases seen as an unproblematic difference. The attempt here to correct even unproblematic differences with reading illustrates how dyslexia can be understood as a part of a machinery of government concerned with fostering as much value as possible from the population. Congenital word-blindness achieved this by identifying bodies in both the populations accredited as normal and as feeble-minded (where more value could be fostered).

The Invention of Congenital Word-blindness as an Event in the History of the Government of Reading

I have demonstrated that the various diagnoses concerned with congenital reading difficulties (congenital word-blindness, amnesia visualis verbalis, congenital alexia) operated as part of various machineries of government that were concerned with proliferating literacy across the body of the population. The goal of imbuing bodies with a certain degree of literacy, even if conventional methods of teaching had failed them, shows that gaining instructions or information from reading printed inscriptions had increased in its importance across the course of the nineteenth and early twentieth centuries. Many of the writers I discussed in the Chapter 7 extolled the benefits of reading (Gray, 1919: 336; Guilfoile, 1921: 131; Schmitt, 1914: 150–1). Their idea of the activity of reading seemed, however, to have been transformed to a more technical activity. Throughout my discussion of a variety of works concerned with the history, philosophy and sociology of reading (Derrida, 1997; Hunter, 1998; Jones and Williamson, 1979; Manguel, 1997; Viswanathan, 1989) and primary sources (Bernard, 1809: 203–4; Hansard, 24 April, 1807, 22 May, 1851; Select Committee of 1816 Education of the Lower Orders in the Metropolis; Stow, 1836) I have suggested that in earlier centuries access to the ability to read and texts themselves was closely guarded, as the potential dangers of a literate population were feared.

As the twentieth century began, new attitudes regarding reading appear to have been developing around the writers associated with the journals *Ophthalmoscope*, *The Psychological Clinic* and *The Elementary School Journal*. In these journals there seems to be consensus regarding the need for literacy to be proliferated throughout the population. I would suggest that the kind of literacy these writers were trying to proliferate throughout the population was different to the dangerous *art* of reading that had long been feared by those who tried to govern others. The kind of literacy that was proliferated throughout the population was the *technique* of reading. While the diagnosis facilitated particular strategies of government, it was imbued with the rationales of the day, concerned with drawing further capital out of the bodies it diagnosed. The reach of strategies of government increased as technologies made more differences visible, producing more complex diagrams of human capabilities, as skills such as reading were marked onto a detailed map of the human mind (Schmitt, 1914: 151).

While congenital word-blindness and its variants were concerned with dispersing literacy throughout the body of the population, the kind of literacy being proliferated was different to the notion of reading that I described in Chapter 3. Although it became important for the population to become literate in the late nineteenth and early twentieth centuries, it was a certain kind of literacy that was being fostered in bodies that had the ability to follow instructions or gain information from printed texts. Reading had become seen as a *technique* rather then as *art*. My discussion in Chapter 3 drew upon Jones and Williamson (1979), Hunter (1988) and Viswanathan (1989) to argue that both the school and the academic study of English literature were technologies concerned with proliferating both literacy and moral values. Congenital word-blindness was also a technology of proliferation, but it was concerned with generating the *technique* of reading. Congenital word-blindness should be understood as an event in the history of reading, a point at which a technology was invented to respond to this shift in the strategy of the government of reading.

I hope to have shown across these pages that diagnostic categories can be considered as technologies of power. Technologies of power augment or shift the flow of power through multifarious mechanisms—be they social, organic or chemical in their make up. The constitution of diagnostic categories to describe specific learning difficulties allows for power to be directed with immense precision onto minute attributes. While the primary concern of this genealogy was to map the formation of the diagnosis of dyslexia, it also allows for an understanding of the increasingly strategic fashion in which power came to flow, as the operations of technologies of power became more discrete in their character.

The Productive Character of Bio-power

The effects of bio-power are, it seems, misunderstood. Despite Foucault's introduction of the concept taking place in the same text where he encouraged his readers to cease to think of the effects of power in negative terms, it is often assumed that Foucault's (and those who follow him) analysis of the animation of bio-power by particular rationalities of government, is negative: that these analyses are concerned with illuminating how a cage-like web of intersecting relations of power multiply and ossify around our bodies, restricting us ever more, imprisoning us. That the production of our bodies is ever more directed and that we are without autonomy, unable to resist. In the first chapter of *Discipline and Punish* Foucault described the imprisonment of the body by the 'modern soul'; a soul crafted and then acted upon by penology, criminology, psychiatry and psychology: 'The soul is the effect and instrument of a political anatomy; the soul is the prison of the body' (1977: 3). It would be straightforward to consider the imprisonment of the body by the soul to be a series of practices concerned with limiting the body. In my view, at least, this is a misunderstanding.

Relations of bio-power, like relations of power in the more general sense, can never be negative, only productive, producing particular bodies and particular populations. The 'modern soul' should perhaps be understood as a refraction of the social, as the culmination of millennia of history acting upon the body in the present. The 'modern soul' acts therefore to produce the conditions in which it is possible for a body to act, or the horizon in which the body can move. The modern soul is understood as imprisoning the body because it produces a mystification, imbuing a body with the sense of having an ahistorical essence. Becoming is replaced by being. In a sense, the soul imprisons the body, as it establishes the conditions through which relations of power can reach through the multitude of human flesh and be articulated onto an individual body. The conditions through which an individual body can resist relations of power and the circumstances that will allow for a body to articulate relations of power onto other bodies are established as the body is endowed with a soul.

So while there is no outside of power, the imprisonment of the body by the soul describes the conditions in which it is possible for power to act on an individual body and the conditions in which it becomes possible to resist power (Revel, 2008). The modern soul becomes a body's ontic reality. As this complexification is reorganised around the body, the residue of the previous relations of power feels like a limit as it becomes apparent that new ways of acting are possible. The soul comes to feel like it imprisons the body when the effects it has had upon the body come to feel static and stationary, while the world changes around it. Genealogy attempts to disturb the mystification of stasis.

In writing this book I understand that it would be possible to view the effects of bio-power I have described as negative. Instead, what is at stake is the description of rationalities of government that have animated relations of bio-power, asking in what ways the flow of power has reacted to this animation, and what kinds of bodies have been produced by the coalescing and intertwining of these relations. Analytical attention has been focused upon how the formation of the diagnostic category and the shifts in uses have increased the size of the population it acted upon. The increase in the size of the population in turn altered the operations it performed as a technology of power.

In my view, one of the greatest strengths of genealogies is the knowledge they offer us of the way that relations of power have been articulated onto us. This genealogy of dyslexia is an attempt to understand the forces that have fashioned the diagnostic category, dyslexia. I believe that attempts to understand the formation of such processes allow us to articulate relations of bio-power *ourselves*, to transform our bodies and the bodies of others. Genealogies therefore act to point out a site upon which relations of power could be animated; they are, in a sense, an attempt to illustrate how individuals have been subjectivated by relations of power, precisely to encourage individuals to take part in their own subjectivation through articulating relations of power onto themselves.

In a sense, this book is a call for individuals and populations to attempt to animate the relations of bio-power that have been articulated onto them, in their own interests rather than according to the perhaps unintended logic of a variety of interwoven rationalities of government. The study has sought to understand the rationalities of government that animate particular relations of bio-power and not to suggest that this is negative, but, alternatively, that the type of bodies these configurations of power have produced were made in the interests of a particular arrangement of rationalities of government. Genealogies are one tactic, one way of resisting the articulation of power onto the body by another. This genealogy has, in one sense, been a way of understanding the weight of relations of power acting upon *my* body, it has been an attempt to understand *how* relations articulated by Hinshelwood, Thomas, Witmer and Orton ultimately affected me—relations of power that act in a complex assemblage upon millions of bodies. I hope that this genealogy will play a modest contribution in allowing for the relations of power that have flowed through the mechanism, provided by the diagnosis of dyslexia, to be understood anew. This book is intended to be part of a strategy for resisting power, for allowing the present, and our present sense of embodiment, to feel less fixed by opening our bodies up to re-constitution through the articulation of bio-power.

Through describing the manner in which a single technology of power interacts and works in conjunction with a diverse machinery of technologies, I hope to have illustrated that over the course of the twentieth century the machinery engaged in subjectivation became more complex in its character. The populations distilled from the multitude of human flesh were be endowed with souls that made visible, and therefore manageable, the most microscopic of human differences. This management is achieved through a peculiar paradox, the proliferation of the visibility of difference also dispersed a kind of homogeneity—the ability to be measured and managed.

Rethinking Genealogy

Nietzsche (1998) inaugurated the genealogical tradition with a topic, the vastness of which was only matched by the brilliance of his analysis—morality. The morality and practices of punishment (1979) became one Foucault's most famous topics in *Discipline and Punish*, and Anglophone writers continued along this trajectory of operating upon smaller topics, which I would refer to as machineries of government, such as psychology (Rose, 1985, 1999), accounting (Miller, 1992, 2001) and statistics (Hacking, 1982, 1990). My application has been to something smaller still, a single diagnostic category, which I have, in turn, considered as a technology of power. This has allowed me to analyse the operation of the diagnosis as a technology that facilitated the flow of power in particular ways, in specific directions and onto carefully chosen bodies.

While there have been previous studies of impairment categories (Davis, 1995, 2008) or disablement (Stiker, 1997) that are strongly influenced by Foucault, this book has attempted to pose questions that derive from genealogy's unique epistemological stance, of which I have then systematically utilised and developed as a genealogical method (detailed in the introduction to this book). The application of the genealogical method to a particular impairment category considering the diagnosis as a technology of power takes a smaller, more precise focus than studies such as Stiker's (1997) that attempted to study the totality of disablement. It is my contention that through writing smaller, precise genealogies of impairment categories, a fuller picture of the history of disablement will be achieved, as the barriers that disabled people face are varied and constantly changing.

Writing genealogies of impairment categories like dyslexia, that were invented to describe particular characteristics problematised by medical professions, educationalists and states over the twentieth century, informs one of the ways in which strategies of government have been diffused into everyday life, reformulating the way that we consider our body's potential capabilities and, indeed, our limitations. Understanding how particular characteristics of individuals and groups become problematised and the processes that lead diagnostic categories to be fashioned is a project that could, of course, be conducted upon a wide variety of impairment categories. Multiple impairment categories need to be analysed in this way if we are to develop further our sociological understanding of what social, economic, political and moral forces problematise certain human characteristics as impairment categories. I would therefore suggest that the methodological approach I have developed in this book should be applied to as broad a collection of impairment categories as possible. It is not just disablement that has its roots in the way a society is organised; the process by which particular human characteristics are problematised and then recognised as impairment categories is also a product of political, moral and economic forces. These values are deeply embedded in the most mundane of daily practices; the crafting of these values by moral, political and economic forces can only be understood through detailed historical work into the practices of experts and the systems of thought they draw upon.

My attempt to develop the genealogical study of impairment categories is intended as a contribution to the development of a *comprehensive* sociology of disablement. It is not an attempt to criticise the social model for excluding impairment, but instead to enrich sociological understandings of disablement by providing a framework for how the formations of particular impairment categories at particular geographical and historical junctures may be studied. Paterson and Hughes (1999) have hitherto called for the sociology of impairment to be focused around the phenomenological study of the body. I, however, would like to offer an alternative approach studying impairment categories through using historical methods of research into the constitution of ways of acting upon the body by particular medical, bureaucratic or lay institutions, rather than as Hughes and Paterson (1997) have done, focusing on the phenomenonological experience of the body.[1] This theoretical focus appears inappropriate as it re-focuses attention upon the individual, which I feel is counter-productive from both a political and sociological point of view.[2] The genealogical method for studying impairment categories that I have developed should thus be distinguished from that of Hughes and Paterson as it focuses on the emergence, development and ossification of impairment categories, rather than on the embodied experience of disabled people.

Considering impairment categories as technologies of power alerts us to the way medical categories are used by physicians and the bureaucratic categories deployed by public bodies to differentiate, sort and act upon people. Impairment categories typically serve as symbols to legitimise a particular service provision, be it bureaucratic, medical, technological or personal support. An impairment category thus functions as a moral value, alerting a particular organisation to the fact that they are obligated to provide certain kinds of support to individuals accredited with the ascribed impairment. Impairment categories should therefore be considered as technologies of government concerned with differentiating people with impairments from the rest of the population. The genealogist here endeavours to be detached, not viewing the object of investigation (an impairment category) as good or bad, but instead as something that cannot be allowed to be seen as a-historical.

One of the conditions of possibility for a diagnosis such as dyslexia was the figurative tool of the norm, a technology as I have detailed that both re-imagined human flesh and how it could be acted on. The great operation that the norm performed was to create universal benchmarks for populations against which individual bodies could be judged. Despite being made possible by the norm, categories such as dyslexia minimised the contours of what was considered normal, adding further and more complex ways in which someone could deviate and therefore become abnormal. As a technology of power, the norm has a tendency to complexify, allowing other technologies to couple with it, producing ways of measuring, assessing and administrating bodies.

The success of the norm as a technology of power no doubt facilitated the growth in the number of dyslexia diagnosis. As I have outlined across the book, the norm allowed for the generalisation of discipline. However, I would now go further and suggest that the norm establishes the disciplinary character of power as the status quo. The norm essentially functions as a benchmark, configuring the individual body to receive the discrete and purposeful touch of power as administrated through the specific operations of technologies that rely on the norm. The norm makes all bodies homogenous in the sense that they can be understood by their degree of deviation from localised norms, while simultaneously making visible an array of differences hitherto unrecognised by the five human senses. The norm transforms human flesh into a calculable body. Diagnoses such as dyslexia were invented within this disciplinary style of thought. These diagnostic categories require the prior intervention of configuring technologies such as the norm to establish the discursive formation in which they will operate. A diagnosis such as this is made technically possible and generalisable onto populations by the prior effects of the technology of power that we call the norm.

For Deleuze and Guattari, segmentation operates in at least three ways: a binary fashion, a circular fashion and a linear fashion. It would seem that the introduction of the norm into the bio-political machinery of government intensifies and accelerates the binary fashion of segmentation in a manner absolutely necessary for the way that capital and bodies were to accumulate over the twentieth century. While it is easy to agree with Deleuze and Guattari that '[t]he human being is a segmentary animal' (1988: 208) it must be noted that the technology of the norm and various disciplines concerned with plotting the human and humanity in numeric terms, augment this process into the diagram of the human, and is best understood as a thousand microscopic attributes plotted onto lines—lines that express the diversity of human capabilities and open these individual human capabilities to management and cultivation. In short, it shows a move from a *material* diagram of humanity to an *immaterial* diagram of humanity, drawn by an array of technical instruments.

Analysing impairment categories as technologies of power and writing their genealogies allows for the conditions that engender the problematisation of particular human differences, and the conditions that produce diagnostic categories that respond to this problematisation to be described. Genealogies of impairment categories are therefore able to shed light upon the character of the specific segmentary logic that problematises human flesh and thus produces impairment categories. Genealogies of impairment categories will help to analyse why some human differences are seen as problematic, while others remain unproblematic.

My conception of a genealogical study of impairment categories builds upon Stone's (1984) study of the 'administrative concept of disability' where:

> The concept of disability is fundamentally the result of political conflict about distributive criteria and the appropriate recipients of social aid. Instead of seeing disability as a set of objective characteristics that render people needy, we can define it in terms of ideas and values about distribution. A political analysis must therefore begin by elucidating the dimensions of the disability concept that give it legitimacy as a distributive criterion. (1984: 172)

Stone is thus conducting a political analysis of the administrative category of 'disabled person'. She provides a lucid analysis of how the administrative category has come to be accepted by particular public and administrative organisations. The genealogical study of impairment categories could, perhaps, have a similar vocation; it must be concerned with how particular impairment categories became legitimised, and explore the moral values, political ideologies and philosophical assumptions that were deployed in this process of legitimisation. It is, simply put, the study of political forces and *how* they have interacted in the construction of a diagnostic or administrative category.

If disablement is a wholly social phenomenon, caused mainly by the organisation of labour along inaccessible and prejudicial lines, then the re-organisation of our working lives, social lives and built environment would eliminate this experience. My belief is that the genealogies of impairment categories produce knowledge concerning how particular impairment categories have been formed by economic, social, bureaucratic and environmental factors. If we are to reorganise our lives to eliminate the disablement that people encounter, we must be attentive to the processes that have caused particular biological and psychological characteristics to be problematised, so that the re-organisation that we engage in does not problematise new sets of characteristics leading to segments of new populations becoming disabled people.

In Chapter 3 I argued that, in conjunction with a shift in the way reading was governed, the relationship between readers and texts has drastically altered with a poetic, or perhaps even spiritual, conception of the activity of reading the book of life (and through doing so unveiling eternal truths) being largely replaced by a conception of reading to gain information. The activity of reading a text became a process through which information was stripped from a page, to be deployed in our work, or providing us with instructions in how to carry out a task. The augmentation of our encounters with texts in day-to-day life seems set to continue if the processes that have occurred during the writing of this book develop further still. Web browsers on smartphones and tablets have added yet another layer of textual engagement with the written word to our lives. While our encounters with texts may be intensifying, the time we have to read texts is shrinking as the pace of life increases. The information bomb described by Paul Virilo (2000) thus becomes a more vital analysis. In 2006 I attended a lecture by Zygmunt Bauman entitled 'Liquid Modern Challenges to Education' (2006). This describes our predicament well, taking up many of the insights that Virilo had initially articulated. Bauman argues that many of us today have free access to a whole host of information at our fingertips—we are able to acquire facts at the touch of button; however, we no longer have the analytical skills to understand it.

It is almost as if the experience of having a difficulty in understanding the printed word is becoming an evasive one in our seemingly literate societies. Schmitt (1914) and Gray (1916c) distinguished between difficulties in 'quality' and 'quantity' in reading; perhaps we are experiencing increasing difficulties in the 'quality' of our reading.

The majority of this book deals with a period that in many ways seems distant. A period in the wake of the industrial revolution when many of the familiar institutions of modern life were forming; it is, however, our contemporary juncture that makes it necessary to return to this period. It would not be controversial to suggest that this articulation of our linguistic capacity into relations of production engendered a mass problematisation of human characteristics. It is this production that I have described throughout this book.

Dyslexia is an impairment category that is seemingly permeated with so many of the significant political rationalities of the twentieth century. In many ways it is emblematic of both the way we laboured and the strategies that governed us. As a diagnosis it formed but a small component of psychology, a machinery of government whose practices and procedures formalised over this period as its influence and prestige grew. As a technology of power, dyslexia acts as a tool of differentiation. It identifies individuals who can be educated, through specific and directed means, differentiating them from a population who had otherwise been considered to be uneducable. The operation that the diagnosis performed (and is still performing) was hospitable to rationalities of government concerned with fostering literacy throughout the population. If we follow Marazzi's assessment, that our economy has undergone a linguistic turn, and the character of our labour has become increasingly communicative and relational, the diagnosis of dyslexia should therefore be understood as a technology that allows for otherwise problematic bodies to be made amenable to the conditions in which they will be required to labour. The rapid increase in the number of people diagnosed with dyslexia signals the potency of psychology as a machinery of government whose practices are articulated into almost every corner of human life. This is arguably the case even more so today considering the rise in cognitive labouring.

Writing this genealogy has uncovered the strange accidents, technological innovations and the political rationalities involved in problematising certain characteristics of a person, as well as how a different set of forces entwined to fashion a impairment category, congenital word-blindness, to describe them. I have become convinced that in the twentieth-first century impairment categories will be fashioned to respond to changing social and economic conditions that we will most likely face. Conducting cartographies of the present (Rose, 2006) that are aware, owing to genealogies like mine, of the economic, political and moral factors that previously crafted impairment categories will, perhaps, offer us some indication of the type of impairment categories we can expect to be formed across the twentieth-first century and the political rationalities that will be involved in their formation.

The blueprint of the machinery that would diagnosis 'dyslexics' may have been fashioned in the late nineteenth century, but its mass deployment occurs later, as the accumulation of capital comes to rely ever more on the immaterial, relational and linguistic capacities of human labour power. This economic shift has the side affect, no doubt, of proliferating diagnostic categories. Increasingly complex human differences can be described and, indeed, managed. As the modes in which human labour becomes increasingly immaterial, so does the diagram of the human. Our attributes, capacities and characteristics are measured and cultivated in ways that surpass the five human senses. I am not denying the existence of biological difference. Rather, the movement of certain differences to the centre of an individual is being affirmed as a result of a particular tactics of power. Power is anterior to the body, it shines upon human flesh, not only making difference visible, but it orders these now visible characteristics, making some salient and positioning others in relative obscurity.

An underlining assertion of the book is that the fashioning of a vast and diverse diagnostic machinery, of which the diagnosis whose genealogy I have described was but a part, accelerated and transformed the way in which bio-power could act upon human flesh, describing and acting upon the body, illustrating a significant shift in how the body was opened up for capitalisation in the twentieth century.

Notes

Chapter 1

1. After surveying much material on dyslexia I have found that these estimates of the numbers of dyslexic diagnoses are all that are available. Significant research still needs to be conducted to understand the various spikes in the number of dyslexia diagnoses over the last 100 years or so.
2. Here I am using bio-politics to refer to the shift in the style of power relations that, according to Foucault (1979), occurred during the nineteenth century, a move from relations of sovereign power to relations of bio-power. I offer a detailed description of literature concerned with this problem in Chapter 2.
3. I am deploying the term government in a Foucauldian sense as not referring to the state but the 'conduct of conduct'. I further elaborate on this concept in Chapter 3.
4. Again, I am using this concept in a Foucauldian manner. A discussion of how I am using this concept is provided in Chapter 3 in the section 'The Technicalities of Governing: Technologies, Government, Governmentality'.
5. My discussion of the norm as a technology of power relies heavily upon Ewald (1990, 1991) and is influenced by Davis (1995).

Chapter 2

1. Maurizio Lazzarato (2002) detailed the need for a distinction.
2. Style is being deployed here in the same sense of Fleck (1981) describes a style of thought.
3. A point that will later be picked up by Hacking (1982, 1990, 1991) and Ewald (1990).

Chapter 3

1. First, Foucault's co-workers and students who were close to him: Donzelot (1979), Castels (1991), Ewald (1990, 1991), Defert (1991), Pasquino (1978, 1991), Procacci (1978, 1998); second, a group of Anglophone writers, some of whom were initially clustered around the journal *Ideology and Consciousness*: Rose (1979, 1984, 1985), Gordon (1991), Hacking (1982, 1990), Miller (1986, 1992), Miller and O'Leary (1987), Burchell (1991), Dean (1994, 1995), Cruikshank (1993, 1994), Hunter (1994) and Valverde (1996).
2. Derrida only makes cursory reference to reading in this long text, spending the majority of his argument describing how speech has been privileged in Western philosophy at the expense of writing.
3. This is likely to be under the influence of a prominent review by Francis Ewald. Foucault here was being presented as having arguments incompatible with Marxism.

4. I am using the term 'break' here in the sense used by Bachelard, Althusser and Foucault from their concept of the epistemological break (Balibar, 1979).

Chapter 4

1. See my discussion in Chapters 3 and 4.

Chapter 5

1. Similar developments were taking place regarding the education of blind children. Reverend Moon and Louis Braille made distinctions between the blind population in general and the 'educatable blind' and 'industrious blind' (Farrrell, 2004: 11).
2. This explains why so many of the earlier cases were diagnosed by ophthalmologists, as this was where parents took their seemingly bright children who had a specific difficulty with reading.
3. Emphasising the localised character of congenital word-blindness has been a feature of all Hinshelwood's writing on word-blindness.
4. A criticism that had already been articulated in the UK by Broadbent (1896) and Hinshelwood (1904).
5. For the same practice see Nettleship (1901), Bruner (1905), Fisher (1905), Thomas (1905), Stephenson (1907, 1910) Claiborne (1906), Jackson (1906) and Ball (1907).
6. This authority can be seen in the continual reference to Hinshelwood's writing across various articles on congenital word-blindness (Nettleship, 1901). He is also one of the view writers of published material in both specialised and general interest journals; his influence thus appears to be wide and far-reaching.

Chapter 8

1. Across several papers, Hughes and Paterson (Hughes, 1999, 2000, 2002; Hughes and Paterson, 1997; Paterson and Hughes, 1999) elaborate what the sociology of impairment would be concerned with and the theoretical traditions it would draw upon—the work draws heavily on phenomenological philosophy, specifically the work of Maurice Merleau-Ponty.
2. I take this to be the case because I side with Norbert Elias (1978) in understanding humans to only exist in groups, never in isolation.

References

Agamben, G. (1995) *Homo Sacer: Sovereign Power and Bare Life* (Standford, CA: Stanford University).

Anderson, C. and Merton, E. (1920a) 'Remedial Work in Reading, Part I', *The Elementary School Journal*, 20(9), 685–701.

Anderson, C. and Merton, E. (1920b) 'Remedial Work in Reading, Part II', *The Elementary School Journal*, 20(10), 772–91.

Anderson, C. and Merton, E. (1921) 'Remedial Work in Silent Reading, Part I', *The Elementary School Journal*, 21(5), 336–48.

Anderson, P. and Meier-Hedde, R. (2001) 'Early Case Reports of Dyslexia in the United States and Europe', *Journal of Learning Disabilities*, 34(1), 9–21.

Bachelard, G. (1984) *The New Scientific Spirit* (Boston, MA: Beacon Press).

Bal, M. (2005) *Reading Rembrandt. Beyond the Word-Image Opposition* (Amsterdam: Amsterdam University Press).

Balibar, È. (1979) 'From Bachelard to Althusser: The Concept of Epistemological Break', *Economy and Society*, 7(3): 24–47.

Ball, M. (1907) 'A Case of Alexia in a Boy of Fifteen', *Annals of Ophthalmology*, 16, 247–8.

Bauman, Z. (1991) *Modernity and Ambivalence* (Cambridge: Polity).

Bauman, Z. (2006) 'Liquid Modern Challenges to Education', https://elgg.leeds.ac.uk/soc6tjw/weblog/1669.html (accessed 15 May 2006).

Bell, A. (1813) *The Madras School, or, Elements of Tuition: Comprising the Analysis of An Experiment in Education, Made at the Male Asylum, Madras; With its Facts, Proofs, and Illustrations: To Which are Added, Extracts of Sermons Preached at Lambeth; A Sketch of a National Institution for Training up the Children of the Poor; And a Specimen of the Mode of Religious Instruction at the Royal Military Asylum, Chelsea* (Edinburgh: Archibald Constable and Co.).

Bell, V. (1993) 'Governing Childhood: Neo-liberalism and the Law', *Economy and Society*, 22(3), 390–405.

Berardi, F. (2009) *Precarious Rhapsody: Semiocapitlaism and the Pathologies of Post-alpha Generation* (London: Minor Compositions).

Bernard, T. (1809) *Of the Education of the Poor: Being the First Part of a Digest of the Reports of the Society for Bettering the Condition of the Poor* (London: Woburn Press).

British Dyslexia Association (2010) 'Latest News', http://www.bdadyslexia.org.uk/news/latest-news.html (accessed 1 October 2010).

Bowden, J. (1911) 'Learning to Read', *The Elementary School Teacher*, 12(1), 21–33.

Bowker, G. C. and Star, S. L. (1999) *Sorting Things Out: Classification and Practice* (Cambridge, MA: MIT Press).

Broadbent, W. (1872) 'Cerebral Mechanisms of Speech and Thought', *Transactions of the Royal Medical and Chirurgical Society*, 55, 145–94.

Broadbent, W. (1896) 'Note on Dr. Hinshelwood's Communication on Word-blindness and Visual Memory', *The Lancet*, 147(3375), 18.

Bruner, W. (1905) 'Congenital Word-blindness', *Ophthalmology: Essays, Abstracts and Review*, 1(2), 189.

Burchell, G. (1991) 'Peculiar Interests: Civil Society and Governing "The System of Natural Liberty"', in Burchell, G., Gordon, C. and Miller, P. (eds) *The Foucault Effect: Studies in Governmentality* (Hemel Hempstead: Harvester Wheatsheaf).

Burchell, G. (1996) 'Liberal Government and Techniques of the Self', in Barry, A., Osborne, T. and Rose, N. (eds) *Foucault and Political Reason: Liberalism Neo-Liberalism and Rationalities of Government* (London: UCL Press).

Butler, J. (2002) 'Bodies and Power, Revisited', *Radical Philosophy*, 114, 13–19.

Canguilhem, G. (1989) *The Normal and Pathological* (New York: Zone Books).

Castels, R. (1991) 'From Dangerousness to Risk', in Burchell, G., Gordon, C. and Miller, P. (eds) *The Foucault Effect: Studies in Governmentality* (Hemel Hempstead: Harvester Wheatsheaf).

Childress, D. (2008) *Johannes Gutenberg and the Printing Press* (Minneapolis, MN: Lerner).

Claiborne, J. (1906) 'Types of Congenital Symbol Amblyopia', *Journal of the American Medical Association*, 47(22), 1813–16.

Compas, B. and Gotlib, I. (2002) *Introduction to Clinical Psychology* (New York: McGraw-Hill Higher Education).

Courtis, S. (1914) 'Standard Tests in English', *The Elementary School Teacher*, 14(8), 374–92.

Cruikshank, B. (1993) 'Revolutions Within: Self-government and Self-esteem', *Economy and Society*, 22(3), 327–44.

Cruikshank, B. (1994) 'The Will to Empower: Technologies of Citizenship and the War on Poverty', *Socialist Review*, 23(4), 29–55.

Cubit, S. (2006) 'Library', *Theory, Culture & Society*, 23(2–3), 591–6.

Davis, L. (1995) *Enforcing Normalcy: Disability, Deafness and the Body* (London, Verso).

Davis, L. (2008) *Obsession: A History* (Chicago, IL: The University of Chicago Press).

Dean, M. (1994) 'The Genealogy of the Gift in Antiquity', *Australian Journal of Anthropology*, 5(3), 320–9.

Dean, M. (1995) 'Governing the Unemployed Self in an Active Society', *Economy and Society*, 24(4), 559–83.

Dean, M. (1999) *Governmentality: Power and Rule in Modern Society* (London: SAGE).

Defert, D. (1991) 'Popular Life' and Insurance Technology. *The Foucault Effect: Studies in Governmentality* (Hemel Hempstead: Harvester Wheatsheaf).

Deleuze, G. (1986) *Nietzsche and Philosophy* (London: Bloomsbury Academic).

Deleuze, G. (1992) *Foucault* (London: Athlone Press).

Deleuze, G. and Guattari, F. (1987) *Anti-Oedipus Capitalism and Schizophrenia Volume 1* (London: Athlone Press).

Deleuze, G and Guattari, F (1988). *A Thousand Plateaus: Capitalism and Schizophrenia Volume 2*. London: Athlone Press

Derrida, J. (1997) *Of Gramatology* (Baltimore, MD: The John Hopkins University Press).

Dillon, M. (1995) 'Sovereignty and Governmentality: From the Problematics of the "New World Order" to the Ethical Problematic of the World Order', *Alternatives*, 20, 323–68.

Donzelot, J. (1979) *The Policing of Families* (London: Hutchinson).

Donzelot, J. (1988) 'The Promotion of the Social', *Economy and Society*, 17(3), 395–427.

Donzelot, J. (1991) 'The Mobilisation of Society', in Burchell, G., Gordon, C. and Miller, P. (eds) *The Foucault Effect: Studies in Governmentality* (Hemel Hempstead: Harvester Wheatsheaf).

Drucker, P. (1969) *The Age of Discontinuity: Guidelines to Our Changing Society* (London: Heinemann).

Elden, S. (2002) 'The War of Races and the Constitution of the State: Foucault's *"Il faut defender la societe"* and the Politics of Calculation', *Boundary 2*, 29(1), 125–51.

Elden, S. (2006) 'National Socialism and the Politics of Calculation', *Social and Cultural Geography*, 7(5), 753–69.

Elias, N. (1978) *What Is Sociology?* (New York: Columbia University Press).

Ewald, F. (1990) 'Norms, Discipline and the Law', *Representations*, April, 138–61.

Ewald, F. (1991) 'Insurance and Risk', in Burchell, G., Gordon, C. and Miller, P. (eds) *The Foucault Effect: Studies in Governmentality* (Hemel Hempstead: Harvester Wheatsheaf).

Ewald, F. (2002) 'The Return of Descartes. Malicious Demon: An Outline of Philosophy of Precaution', in Baker, T. and Simon, J. (eds) *Embracing Risk: The Changing Culture of Insurance and Responsibility*, pp. 273–301 (Chicago, IL: Chicago University Press).

Farrell, M. (2004) *Special Educational Needs: A Resource for Practitioners* (London: SAGE).

Fildes, L. (1921) 'A Psychological Inquiry into the Nature of the Condition Known as Congenital Word-blindness', *Brain*, 44(3), 286–307.

Fisher, J. H. (1905) 'Case of Congenital Word Blindness (Inability to Learn to Read)', *Ophthalmological Review*, 24, 315–18.

Fleck, L. (1981) *Genesis and Development of a Scientific Fact* (Chicago, IL: University of Chicago Press).

Ford, C. (1928) 'A Case of Congenital Word-Blindness Showing its Social Implications', *The Psychological Clinic*, 17(1), 73–84.

Foucault, M. (1977) *Discipline and Punish: the Birth of the Prison* (London: Allen Lane).

Foucault, M. (1979) *The History of Sexuality, Vol. 1. An Introduction* (London: Allen Lane).

Foucault, M. (1980) 'Truth and power', in *Power/Knowledge, Selected Interviews and Other Writings 1972–1977* (New York: Pantheon Books).

Foucault, M. (1989a) *The Archaeology of Knowledge* (London: Routledge).

Foucault, M. (1989b) *The Birth of the Clinic* (London: Routledge).

Foucault, M. (1991) 'Politics and the Study of Discourse', in Burchell, G., Gordon, C. and Miller, P. (eds) *The Foucault Effect: Studies in Governmentality* (Chicago, IL: University of Chicago Press).

Foucault, M. (1997a) 'What is Enlightenment?', in *Ethics. Essential Works of Foucault, 1954–1984*, Vol. I (Middlesex: Penguin Books).

Foucault, M. (1997b) 'On The Genealogy of Ethics', in *Ethics. Essential Works of Foucault, 1954–1984*, Vol. I (Middlesex: Penguin Books).

Foucault, M. (1997c) 'Sex, Power, and the Politics of Identity', in *Ethics. Essential Works of Foucault, 1954–1984*, Vol. I (Middlesex: Penguin Books).

Foucault, M. (1998a) 'Nietzsche, Genealogy, History', in *Aesthetics. Essential Works of Foucault, 1954–1984*, Vol. II (Middlesex: Penguin Books).

Foucault, M. (1998b) 'Structuralism and Post-structuralism', in *Aesthetics. Essential Works of Foucault, 1954–1984*, Vol. II (Middlesex: Penguin Books).

Foucault, M. (1998c) 'Life: Experience and Science', in *Aesthetics. Essential Works of Foucault, 1954–1984*, Vol. II (Middlesex: Penguin Books).

Foucault, M. (2000a) 'Truth and Juridical Forms', in *Power. Essential Works of Foucault, 1954–1984*, Vol. III (Middlesex: Penguin Books).

Foucault, M. (2000b) 'Questions of Method', in *Power. Essential Works of Foucault, 1954–1984*, Vol. III (Middlesex: Penguin Books).

Foucault, M. (2000c) 'Useless to Revolt', in *Power. Essential Works of Foucault, 1954–1984*, Vol. III (Middlesex: Penguin Books).

Foucault, M. (2000d) 'Governmentality', in *Power. Essential Works of Foucault, 1954–1984*, Vol. III (Middlesex: Penguin Books).

Foucault, M. (2001) *Fearless Speech* (Los Angeles, CA: Semiotexte).

Foucault, M. (2003) *Society Must be Defended: Lectures at the Collège de France 1975–1976* (New York: Palgrave Macmillan).

Foucault, M. (2006) *History of Madness* (London: Routledge).

Foucualt, M. (2007) *Security, Territory, Population: Lectures at the Collège de France 1977–1978* (New York: Palgrave Macmillan).

Foucault, M. (2008) *The Birth of Biopolitics: Lectures at the Collège de France 1977–1978* (New York: Palgrave Macmillan).

Foucault, M. (2010) *The Government of the Self and Others: Lectures at the Collège de France 1982–1983* (New York: Palgrave Macmillan).

Garland-Thomson, R. (1997) *Extraordinary Bodies: Figuring Physical Disability in American Culture and Literature* (New York: Columbia University Press).

Giddens, A. (1999) 'Risk and Responsibility', *Modern Law Review*, 62(1), 1–10.

Gieryan, T. (1983) 'Boundary-work and the Demarcation of Science from Non-science: Strains and Interests in Professional Ideologies of Scientists', *American Sociological Review*, 48(6), 781–95.

Glatzer, N. (1974) *I Am a Memory Come Alive: Autobiographical Writings of Franz Kafka* (New York: Schocken Books).

Gordon, C. (1991) 'Introduction', in Burchell, G., Gordon, C. and Miller, P. (eds) *The Foucault Effect: Studies in Governmentality* (Hemel Hempstead: Harvester Wheatsheaf).

Gray, W. (1916a) 'Reading in the Elementary Schools of Indianapolis', *The Elementary School Journal*, 19(5), 336–53.

Gray, W. (1916b) 'Methods of Testing Reading', *The Elementary School Journal*, 16(5), 231–46.

Gray, W. (1916c) 'Methods of Testing Reading II', *The Elementary School Journal*, 16(6), 281–98.

Gray, W. (1919) 'Reading in the Elementary Schools of Indianapolis', *The Elementary School Journal*, 19(5), 336–53.

Guattari, F. and Alliez, E. (1996) *Capitalist Systems, Systems, Structures and Processes. The Guattari Reader* (Cambridge, MA: Blackwell).

Guilfoile, E. (1921) 'Using the Public Library in the Teaching of Reading', *The Elementary School Journal*, 22(2), 126–31.

Hacking, I. (1982) 'Bio-Power and the Avalanche of Printed Numbers', *Humanities in Society*, 5, 279–95.

Hacking, I. (1990) *The Taming of Chance* (Cambridge: Cambridge University Press).

Hacking, I. (1991) 'How Should We Do the History of Statistics?', in Burchell, G., Gordon, C. and Miller, P. (eds) *The Foucault Effect: Studies in Governmentality* (Hemel Hempstead: Harvester Wheatsheaf).

Hansen, R. and King, D. (2001) 'Eugenic Ideas, Political Interests, and Policy Variance Immigration and Sterilization Policy in Britain and the US', *World Politics*, 53(2), 237–63.

Hansard (1807) 'Parliamentary Debates (series 1)', Vol. 9, 24 April, 538–50.

Hansard (1851) 'Parliamentary Debates (series 4)', Vol. 116, 22 May, 1279.

Hasian, M. (1996) *The Rhetoric of Eugenics in Anglo-American Thought* (Athens, GA: University of Georgia Press).

Heidegger, M. (1977) *The Question Concerning Technology and Other Essays* (New York: Harper Torchbooks).

Henriques, J. (1984). *Changing the Subject: Psychology, Social Regulation and Subjectivity* (London: Routledge).

Hinshelwood, J. (1895) 'Word-blindness and Visual Memory', *Lancet*, 2, 1564–570.

Hinshelwood, J. (1896) 'A Case of Dyslexia a Peculiar Form of Word-blindness', *The Lancet* 1451–4.

Hinshelwood, J. (1900a) 'Congenital Word-blindness', *The Lancet*, 1, 1506–8.

Hinshelwood, J. (1900b) *Mind, Letter and Word-blindness* (London: Lewis & Co.).

Hinshelwood, J. (1902) 'Congenital Word-blindness, With Reports of Two Cases', *Ophthalmic Review*, 21(246), 91–9.

Hinshelwood, J. (1904) 'A Case of Congenital Word-blindness', *Ophthalmoscope*, 2(10), 399–405.

Hinshelwood, J. (1907) 'Four Cases of Congenital Word-blindness Occurring in the Same Family', *British Medical Journal*, 2(2444), 1229–53.

Hinshelwood, J. (1912) 'The Treatment of Word-blindness, Acquired and Congenital', *British Medical Journal*, 2, 1033–5.

Hook, D. (2001) 'Discourse, Knowledge, Materiality, History: Foucault and Discourse Analysis', *Theory Psychology*, 11(4), 521–47.

Hughes, B. (1999) 'The Constitution of Impairment: Modernity and the Aesthetic of Oppression', *Disability and Society*, 14(2), 155–72.

Hughes, B. (2000) 'Medicine and the Aesthetic Invalidation of Disabled People', *Disability and Society*, 15(4), 555–68.

Hughes, B. (2002) 'Bauman's Strangers: Impairment and the Invalidation of Disabled People in Modern and Post-modern Cultures', *Disability and Society*, 17(5), 325–40.

Hughes, B. and Paterson, K. (1997) 'The Social Model of Disability and the Disappearing Body: Towards a Sociology of Impairment', *Disability and Society*, 12(3), 325–40.

Hunter, I. (1988) *Culture and Government* (London: Macmillan).

Hunter, I. (1994) *Rethinking the School: Subjectivity, Bureaucracy, Criticism* (Sydney: Allen and Unwin).

Hunter, I. (1998) 'Uncivil Society: Liberal Government and the Deconfessionalisation of Politics', in Dean, M. and Hindess, B. (eds) *Governing Australia: Studies in Contemporary Rationalities of Government* (Melbourne: Cambridge University Press).

Jackson, E. (1906) 'Developmental Alexia (Congenital Word Blindness)', *American Journal of Medial Sciences*, 131, 843–8.

Jacyna, S. (1994) 'Construing Silence: Narrative of Language Loss in early Nineteenth-Century France', *Journal of the History of Medicine and Allied Science*, 49(3), 333–61.

Jacyna, S. (2000) *Lost Words. Narrative of Language and the Brain 1825–1926* (Princeton, NJ: Princeton University Press).

Jones, K. and Williamson, K. (1979) 'The Birth of the Schoolroom', *Ideology and Consciousness*, 5, 59–110.

Judd, C. (1914) 'Reading Tests', *The Elementary School Teacher*, 14(8), 365–73.

Kearins, K. and Hooper, K. (2002) 'Genealogical Method and Analysis', *Accounting, Auditing & Accountability Journal*, 15(5), 733–57.

Kendal, G. and Wickham, G. (1999) *Using Foucault's Methods* (London: SAGE).

Klossowski, P. (2000) 'Nietzshce and the Vicious Circle', (London: Continuum).

Kussmaul, A. (1877) 'Diseases of the Nervous System and Disturbances of Speech', in von Ziemensen, H. (ed.) and McCreey, J. A. (trans.) *Cyclopeida of the Practice of Medicine*, pp. 770–8 (New York: William Wood).

Larner, W. and Walters, W. (2004) 'Globalization as Governmentality', *Alternatives: Global, Local, Political*, 29, 495–514.

Lazzarato, M. (1996) *Immaterial Labour. Radical Thought in Italy: A Potential Politics*, pp. 133–47 (Minneapolis, MN: University of Minnesota Press).

Lazzarato, M. (2002) 'From Biopower to Biopolitics', *PLI: Warwick Journal of Philosophy*, 13, 99–110.

Lotringer, S. and Marazzi, C. (2007) *Autonomia: Post-Political Politics* (Cambridge, MA: MIT Press).

McCready, E. (1925) 'The Aphasias of Childhood Congenital Word-Blindness and Word-Deafness as Causes of Mental Retardation and Deviation', *Southern Medical*, 18(9), 635–46.

Manguel, A. (1997) *A History of Reading* (Kent: Flamingo).

Marazzi, C., Hardt, M. and Conti, G. (2008) *Capital and Language: From the New Economy to the War Economy* (Los Angeles, CA: Semiotext).

Marazzi, C. (2011a) 'Dyslexia and the Economy', *Angelaki*, 16(3), 19–32.

Marazzi, C. (2011b) *Capital and Affects: The Politics of the Language Economy* (Los Angeles, CA: Semiotext).

Marx, K. (1974) *Economic and Philosophic Manuscripts of 1844* (Moscow: Progress Publishers).

Miller, P. (1986) 'Psychotherapy of Work and Unemployment', in Miller, P. and Rose, N. (eds) *The Power of Psychiatry* (Cambridge: Polity Press).

Miller, P. (1992) 'Accounting and Objectivity: The Invention of Calculating Selves and Calculable Spaces', *Annals of Scholarship*, 9(1/2), 61–86.

Miller, P. (2001) 'Governing by Numbers: Why Calculative Practices Matter', *Social Research*, 68(2), 379–96.

Miller, J. (1993) *The Passion of Michel Foucault* (Boston, MA: Harvard University Press).

Miller, P. and O'Leary, T. (1987) 'Accounting and the Construction of the Governable Person', *Accounting, Organizations and Society*, 12(3), 235–65.

Miller, P. and Rose, N. (1990) 'Governing Economic Life', *Economy and Society*, 17(2), 1–31.

Minogue, B. (1927) 'Congenital Word Blindness a Case Study', *Psychiatric Quarterly*, 1(2), 226–30.

Morgan, P. (1896) 'A Case of Congenital Word Blindness', *British Medical Journal*, 2(2), 1378.

Mucchielli, R. (1963) *La dyslexie, maladie du siècle* (Paris: Les Editions Sociales Francaises).

Nettleship, E. (1901) 'Cases of Congenital Word-blindness (Inability to Learn to Read)', *Ophthalmic Review,* 20(233), 61–7.

Nietzsche, F. (1998) *On the Genealogy of Morality: A Polemic* (Indianapolis, IN: Hackett Publishing).

O'Malley, P. (2000) 'Configurations of Risk', *Economy and Society,* 29(4), 45–59.

Orton, S. T. (1925) '"Word-blindness" in school children', *Archives of Neurology and Psychiatry,* 14, 285–516.

Osborne, T. (1993) 'On Liberalism, Neo-liberalism and the "Liberal Profession" of Medicine', *Economy and Society,* 26(4), 345–56.

Osborne, T. (1997) 'Of Health and Statecraft', in Petersen, A. and Bunton, R. (eds) *Foucault, Health and Medicine* (London: Routledge).

Pasquino, P. (1978) '*Theatricum Politicum.* The Genealogy of Capital: Police and the State of Prosperity', *Ideology and Consciousness,* 4, 41–5.

Pasquino, P. (1991) 'Theatrum Politicum: The Genealogy of Capital—Police and the State of Prosperity', in Burchell, G., Gordon, C. and Miller, P. (eds) *The Foucault Effect: Studies in Governmentality* (Hemel Hempstead: Harvester Wheatsheaf).

Paterson, K. and Hughes, B. (1999) 'Disability Studies and Phenomenology the Carnal Politics of Everyday Life', *Disability and Society,* 14(5), 597–610.

Petersen, A. (1997) 'Risk, Governance and the New Public Health', in Petersen, A. and Bunton, R. (eds) *Foucault, Health and Medicine,* pp. 189–206 (London: Routledge).

Philips, B. (1990) *School Psychology at a Turning point* (San Francisco: Jossey-Bass Publishers).

Porter, T. M. (1986) *The Rise of Statistical Thinking, 1820–1990* (Princeton, NJ: Princeton University Press).

Procacci, G. (1978) 'Social Economy and the Government of Poverty', *Ideology and Consciousness,* 4, 55–72.

Procacci, G. (1998) 'Poor Citizens: Social Citizenship and the Crisis of the Welfare State', in Hännimen, S. (ed.) *The Displacement of Social Polices* (Jväskylä: SoPhi).

Rabinow, P. and Rose, N. (2006) 'Biopower Today', *Biosocieties,* 1(2), 195–217.

Revel, J. (2008) 'The Materiality of the Immaterial: Foucault, Against the Return', *Radical Philosophy,* 149.

Rich, E. (1970) *The Education Act 1870: A Study of Public Opinion* (Harlow: Longmans).

Rose, N. (1979) 'The Psychological Complex: Mental Measurement and Social Administration', *Ideology and Consciousness,* 5, 5–68.

Rose, N. (1984) *The Birth of Individual Psychology in England, 1870–1939,* PhD Thesis, University of London Institute of Education.

Rose, N. (1985) *The Psychological Complex: Psychology, Politics and Society in England 1869–1939* (London: Routledge & Kegan Paul).

Rose, N. (1987) 'Beyond the Public/Private Division: Law, Power and the Family', *Journal of Law and Society,* 1, 61–76.

Rose, N. (1991) 'Governing by Numbers: Figuring out Democracy', *Accounting, Organizations and Society,* 16(7), 673–92.

Rose, N. (1993) 'Government, Authority and Expertise in Advanced Liberalism', *Economy and Society,* 22(3), 283–99.

Rose, N. (1996a) 'The Death of the Social? Re-figuring the Territory of Government', *Economy and Society,* 25(3), 327–56.

Rose, N. (1996b) 'Governing "Advanced" Liberal Democracies', in Barry, A., Osborne, T. and Rose, N. (eds) *Foucault and Political Reason: Liberalism, Neo-Liberalism and rationalities of Government* pp. 37–64 (London: UCL Press).

Rose, N. (1999) *Governing the Soul: The Shaping of the Private Self* (London, Free Association Books).

Rose, N. (2001) 'The Politics of Life Itself', *Theory, Culture and Society*, 18(6), 1–30.

Rose, N. (2006) *The Politics of Life Itself: Biomedicine, Power, and Subjectivity in the Twenty-First Century* (Princeton, NJ: Princeton University Press).

Rose, N. and Miller, P. (1992) 'Political Power Beyond the State: Problematic of Government', *British Journal of Sociology*, 43(2), 173–205.

Rutherford, W. (1909) 'The Aetiology of Congenital Word-blindness With an Example', *British Journal Children Diseases*, 6, 484–8.

Schmitt, C. (1914) 'School Subjects as Material for Tests of Mental Ability', *The Elementary School Journal*, 15(3), 150–61.

Schmitt, C. (1915) "Standardization of Tests for Defective Children', *The Psychological Monographs*, 19(3), i–181.

Schmitt, C (1918a) 'Developmental Alexia: Congenital Word-Blindness, or Inability to Learn to Read', *The Elementary School Journal*, 18(9), 680–700.

Schmitt, C. (1918b) 'Developmental Alexia: Congenital Word-Blindness, or Inability to Learn to Read—*Concluded*', *The Elementary School Journal*, 18(10), 757–69.

Select Committee (1816) 'Education of the Lower Orders in the Metropolis', *Parliamentary Papers*, IV.

Stephenson, S. (1907). 'Six Cases of Congenital Word-blindness Affecting Three Generations of One Family', *Ophthalmoscope*, 5, 482–4.

Stephenson, S. (1910) 'Review of Current Literature Congenital Word-blindness', *The Ophthalmoscope*, 8(1), 30–1.

Stiker, H. (1997) *A History of Disability* (Ann Arbor, MI: University of Michigan Press).

Stone, D. (1984) *The Disabled State* (Philadelphia, PA: Temple University Press).

Stow, D. (1836) *The Training System Adopted in the Model Schools of the Glasgow Educational Society a Manual for Infant and Juvenile Schools, Which Includes a System of Moral Training Suited to the Condition of Large Towns* (Glasgow: M'Phun).

Thomas, C.J. (1905) 'Congenital Word Blindness and its Treatment', *Ophthalmoscope*, 3, 380.

Toscano, A. (2008) 'In Praise of Negativism', in O'Sullivan, S. and Zepke, S. (eds) *Deleuze, Guattari, and the Production of the New* (London: Continuum).

Town, C. (1911) 'Congenital Aphasia', *The Psychological Clinic*, 5, 167–79.

Valverde, M. (1996) '"Despotism" and ethical governance', *Economy and Society*, 25(3), 357–72.

Virilio, P. (2000) *The Information Bomb* (London: Verso).

Virno, P. (2003) *A Grammar of the Multitude: An Analysis of Contemporary Forms of Life* (Los Angeles, CA: Semiotexte).

Viswanathan, G. (1989) *Masks of Conquest: Literary Study and British Rule in India* (New York: Columbia University Press).

Volkman, H. and Noble, I. (1915) 'Retardation as Indicated by One Hundred City School Reports', *The Psychological Clinic*, 7, 75–81.

Waldo, K. (1915) 'Tests in Reading in Sycamore Schools', *The Elementary School Journal*, 15(15), 251–68.

Westergaard, H. (1932) *Contributions to the History of Statistics* (London: PS King & Son).

Witmer, L. (1896) 'Practical Work in Psychology', *Paediatrics*, 2, 462–71.

Witmer, L. (1897) 'The Organization of Practical Work in Psychology', *Psychological Review*, 4, 116.

Witmer, L. (1907a) 'Clinical Psychology', *The Psychological Clinic*, 1(1), 1–9.

Witmer, L. (1907b) 'A Case of Chronic Bad Spelling, Amnesia Visualis Verbalis', *The Psychological Clinic*, 1(1), 53–64.

Witmer, L. (1913) 'Children with mental Defects Distinguished from Mentally Defective Children', *The Psychological Clinic*, 7, 173–81.

Witmer, L. (1916) 'Congenital Aphasia and Feeblemindedness—A Clinical Diagnosis', *The Psychological Clinic*, 10, 181–91.

Witmer, L. (1919) 'The Raining of Very Bright Children', *The Psychological Clinic*, 13(1919), 88–96.

Witmer, L. (1922) 'Intelligence—A Definition', *The Psychological Clinic*, 14, 65–7.

Index